Positive Ethics for Mental Health Professionals

A Proactive Approach

Positive Ethics for Mental Health Professionals

A Proactive Approach

Second Edition

Sharon K. Anderson
Colorado State University

Mitchell M. Handelsman
University of Colorado Denver

WILEY Blackwell

To my adult kids, I appreciate and love you more than you can know.

To my mentor, Karen Kitchener and my students who have challenged my thinking.

To Jesus, my best teacher.

Sharon

To my wife Debbi, with whom I will now have more time to spend—promise!

To all my teachers, including all my students.

To the memory of my parents, whose many gifts to me included an appreciation for education and the people involved in it.

Mitch

"I thought ethics would be arduous and full of technical terms and rules... This book was transformative in the way I look at ethics. It was so easy to read/understand and the layout made it so relatable. I really appreciate the Journal Entry prompts and the Food for Thought prompts as well! Who knew I would find an ethics book I couldn't put down?!"

A. E.
First-Year Counseling Psychology Graduate Student
University of Santa Clara

Contents

About the Authors

Sharon K. Anderson, Ph.D., is Professor of Counseling and Career Development at Colorado State University. In 1993, Sharon earned her Ph.D. in Counseling Psychology from the University of Denver. Sharon became a licensed psychologist in 1995. Her experience as a practitioner includes private practice with adults and older people, supervision of masters-level students and those seeking licensure, and consultation regarding ethical issues in practice. Sharon has taught the master's-level ethics course for counseling students for over 25 years—teaching/mentoring a multitude of students. She has co-authored or co-edited other ethics books used by psychologists (*Foundations of Ethical Practice, Research and Teaching in Psychology and Counseling*) and life coaches (*Law and Ethics in Coaching: How to Solve and Avoid Difficult Problems in Your Practice*). She has over 50 publications including books, book chapters, and refereed articles, most of them looking at the practice of professional ethics, teaching ethics, and issues of privilege. In her spare time she rides her motorcycle, reads for enjoyment and rejuvenation, and travels to see family.

Mitchell M. Handelsman, Ph.D., is Professor of Psychology and CU President's Teaching Scholar at the University of Colorado Denver, where he has been since 1982. Mitch earned his Ph.D. from the University of Kansas in 1981. He is a licensed psychologist and a Fellow of the American Psychological Association (STP). He served for a year (1989–1990) in Washington DC as an APA Congressional Science Fellow. Mitch has won numerous teaching awards, including the 1992 CASE (Council for the Advancement and Support of Education) Colorado Professor of the Year Award, and STP's Excellence in Teaching Award in 1995. He has co-authored one other ethics book, *Ethical Dilemmas in Psychotherapy: Positive Approaches to Decision Making* (2015; with Sam Knapp and Michael Gottlieb). He is an associate editor of the *APA Handbook of Ethics in Psychology* (2012). He has published over 70 refereed articles and book chapters, many on ethics- and teaching-related topics. His blog for *PsychologyToday.com* ("The Ethical Professor") focuses on ethical and teaching issues. He is co-author of *The Life of Charlie Burrell: Breaking the Color Barrier in Classical Music*. In his spare time he plays jazz trumpet.

Preface

Welcome to our second edition!

Becoming an ethical psychotherapist or counselor is more than memorizing rules—it is a journey. We wrote this book to help students and practitioners navigate this journey towards a professional identity in a way that integrates their personal ethics and values with the professional ethics and traditions of psychotherapy and counseling.

From the feedback we received, readers found the first edition, engaging positive in its approach, and respectful of their backgrounds. We invite readers to become active explorers, not passive recipients of disembodied rules and laws.

In our second edition, we have kept the format and approach of the first edition. We still present a variety of discussions, case scenarios, thought exercises, and writing assignments. These are meant to (a) introduce readers to all the major ethical issues in psychotherapy, including boundaries, confidentiality, informed consent, supervision, and terminating therapy; (b) help readers explore their core, which includes personal needs, motivations, and values; (c) encourage readers to understand the rational and irrational aspects of ethical thinking and decision making; (d) address with readers issues of social responsibility and cultural awareness; and (e) encourage readers to take a proactive and preventive approach to applying ethics to every facet of their professional behavior.

Within this basic structure, however, we have made some important changes in the second edition. We have expanded our discussion of social responsibility. We have paid more attention to how real professionals make real decisions, including discussions of cognitive and other errors (we call these *tripping points*) that psychotherapists confront in their choice-making process. Finally, we have updated the content and literature cited in the book, including new content around ethics and technology.

Like the first edition, this second edition can be used as a primary or ancillary text for ethics courses in all the mental health fields. Instructors can use it as a supplemental text for courses in professional issues, psychotherapy methods, counseling theories and techniques, and survey courses in clinical and counseling psychology, social work, counseling, and marital and family therapy.

Because this book focuses on the basic aspects of professional ethical identity and ethical reasoning skills, it will be useful to readers over time as they re-adjust their professional identities in reaction to inevitable changes in life situations, professional positions, laws/regulations, and ethics codes.

We also wrote this book to help us teach our own courses, and for our fellow instructors who may be new to teaching ethical issues as an entire course or part of a course. Instructors will find that they can organize class discussions and assignments around the exercises and vignettes from the chapters, or they can use the book to supplement their own methods and materials.

We wish to thank many people who have been involved in the long journey we've taken since our initial conversations about an ethics book. Our agent, Neil Salkind of Studio B, who was instrumental in helping us conceive of this book in its present form and encouraging us to undertake the project; our first edition editor Christine Cardone; our current editor Darren Lalonde and associate managing editor Monica Rogers; Sam Knapp and Michael Gottlieb for their essential work on the ethical acculturation model; and Allison Bashe for her work on the ethics autobiography. We'd like to recognize the following people have provided valuable assistance and feedback to us regarding previous iterations of the book: Tamar Ares, Bill Briggs, Pam Daniel, Pam Fritzler, Sharon Hamm, Susan Heitler, Mark Kirchhofer, Teresa Kostenbauer, Margie Krest, Amos Martinez, Natalie Meinerz, Amber Reed, and Deb Wescott.

Any imperfections that remain in the book, of course, are our responsibility alone.

Introduction

The Mansion of Psychotherapy and the Staircase of Ethics

Picture this: You enter a wonderful mansion. It is over a century old, but clearly is in the process of continual modernization, upgrading, and renovation. However, it retains lots of its traditional luster and elegance. As the mansion has been upgraded and the surrounding neighborhoods have expanded, the mansion has come to fit in and contribute to the community. Although parts of the mansion always need repair, it is the place you have dreamed about since you were much younger. No matter how much time you've already spent in the mansion, you are still working on feeling welcome and at home.

From the foyer, you can catch glimpses of the many rooms in the mansion, on many different levels. From this view, some look brand new and others look somewhat familiar, like rooms in other places you've been in your life. They might even contain some furniture from your previous houses. One thing is for sure: No matter how many times you visit the different rooms, they seem to change over time. Thus, you continually need to re-acquaint yourself with the rooms.

The only way to get to the rooms is via an immense and complex spiral staircase that moves in and out of the various rooms at various levels. Like the mansion and the neighborhood in which it sits, the staircase keeps changing and is a challenge to climb. At places the staircase has railings and is well lit, but this is not the case everywhere. Some parts of the staircase are downright treacherous, especially if you're not paying attention. You notice some steps are not level; they might be slippery or have imperfections that make tripping easy. You get the impression that some folks who've spent more time in the mansion than you have traversed the staircase without much concern. But upon closer inspection you find that even the long-timers get tripped up—sometimes on the most familiar parts of the staircase going to the most familiar rooms. You, like all who enter the mansion, are naturally prone to trip up at times while navigating the stairs. The fact that, at times, the staircase is uneven, inadequately lit, with handrails missing, makes the navigation fraught with some anxiety. You might wonder, "Can I do this? Can I (continue to) climb this staircase to visit all the rooms?"

Sometimes you're so motivated to get to a particular room that you want to skip a step, and sometimes these steps you want to skip are the very ones you need to step on to prepare for the next step and the rooms you want to enter. Sometimes you forget what floor you're on. Sometimes you even forget that there are stairs! You know that climbing the stairs, which is so rewarding, takes effort and persistence. No matter where you are on the staircase, there are more stairs, more rooms to explore, and more spectacular views. What a beautiful mansion to be in!

The metaphor, like any metaphor, is not perfect. The mansion represents you and the profession. You can see the mansion with its staircase and rooms of furniture as the totality of you in the profession. This is where you now live as a developing, or seasoned, psychotherapist. The different rooms represent aspects of you and the profession. Some rooms represent you—your values, needs, motivations, and so forth—and other rooms represent the culture of the profession— its values, traditions, processes, skills, knowledge, and ethics. Many rooms, of course, are furnished and decorated with both personal and professional things. The mansion, then, includes your personal identity and your (new) professional home.

The steps on the spiral staircase represent the process of making ethical decisions and choices. As such, it is a big part of developing your professional identity—making your way in the profession. The choices involve small individual behaviors and broad aspects of what it means to be a therapist or counselor. The staircase connects the elements of yourself—your core—and the profession that allow you to function, both effectively and ethically.

We want to join you, wherever you are on the staircase, on your climb to the next room and/or the next level of the mansion. We will help you navigate the staircase and explore the rooms by sharing observations, stories, information, and questions. So, think of this book as a dialogue between you and us. If we're successful, you will be better able to understand what it takes to navigate the spiral staircase and anticipate the tripping points and joys of your continued ascent and your entry into the different rooms. You will know what is important to you—your core—and what is important about ethics and ethical (a) identity, (b) thinking and choice making, (c) tripping points, and (d) behaviors.

Before we proceed to three important themes, we need to talk about some terms.

Some Terminology

We want to create a common understanding of some terminology. When people write about morals and ethics in philosophy, mental health, medicine, and other fields, they define the words "moral" and "ethical" in a myriad of ways. Some authors use the two terms synonymously; others give them very specific and different meanings. Both terms refer to judgments of right and wrong behavior and the justifications we make for those judgments. In this book we will use the term "ethics" when we refer to professional behaviors, judgments, and decisions. We will use "personal ethics" when we refer to personal beliefs about right and wrong, and "morals" when we are referring to a wider range of behaviors, judgments, and decisions, including those in personal relationships.

Behaving ethically by following rules to avoid punishment has been termed *remedial ethics* (Knapp et al., 2017). We are all for avoiding punishment, but behaving ethically is not only a matter of following rules—although your professional career might go better when you do. We believe that professionals are motivated to do good work and actualize their highest moral and ethical selves—coming from their core or essential self. Here we are talking about *positive ethics* (Handelsman et al., 2009), which is the study of ethics that includes higher levels of motivation and behavior. Focusing on positive themes, the ethical ideal, is more effective, more professionally sustaining, and more fun than focusing only on rules and what we shouldn't do (Handelsman et al., 2009; Knapp et al., 2017). At the same time, we aren't talking about perfection. Perfection is way overrated and impossible. We are human and bound to make ethical mistakes and missteps. What we do at times like these is what matters (Welfel, 2016).

We're going to talk a lot about our professional and ethical identities. We will use the terms synonymously, or put a slash between them, because we believe that ethics is such a big part of our professional identity that there is no real difference between the two. Professional/ethical identities are at the heart of good therapy practice, good supervision, and good relationships with other professionals.

What does professional/ethical identity mean? Researchers and experts offer a variety of ideas. Some see professional/ethical identity as an integration between the person and the professional commitment to ethics (Monson & Hamilton, 2010). Lloyd-Hazlett and Foster (2017) describe it as the amount of integration across the counselor's "personal and professional ethical commitments" (p. 91). Auxier et al. (2003) see the counselor's ethical identity as one of combining the personal, which includes values and morals, with the professional, which includes roles and decisions. For us, ethical identity is this view of self as an ethical person. Drawing from Blasi (1984) and his understanding of identity, we understand that ethical identity and professional/ethical identity includes this "organization of self-related information" that holds ethical thinking, behavior/choices, and a sense of integrity (congruence and consistency of who one is) as key or critical to continue to be the person and the professional they are (Anderson, 2015).

Mental health professionals use a variety of terms to describe what they do—the two major terms being psychotherapy and counseling. In the interest of clarity and brevity, we will use the terms counseling, psychotherapy, and therapy interchangeably.

Developing and Exploring Your Moral and Professional/ Ethical Identity

No matter where we are in our career and our development, we can uncover, explore, and articulate deeper aspects of our being … the core of our identity. Our core includes our motivations, needs, values, emotions, social identities, and personal morals (Anderson, 2015; Blasi, 1984).

Our professional/ethical identities likely develop out of our core in a cyclical (spiral!) fashion rather than in a straight line. We discover parts of our core identity, and that influences how we view the profession's culture and our commitment to ethics. In turn, the experience of our profession's ethics and culture influences who we are at our core.

Sharon recalls two examples that highlight this spiral of personal and professional influence:

> Many years ago an advisee scheduled an appointment with me. I thought our discussion would be about her upcoming classes. I was very wrong: She came into my office and announced she no longer saw herself fitting well with the counseling profession's ethical culture—she was going to pursue a different career where her personal values and ethics were a better match with the profession. Through exploring what was in her core, she was clear that some of her personal values were non-negotiable. She was very committed to some of her personal values and morals and didn't know how she would keep those from being part of her work. For example, she didn't agree with abortion and knew that as a high school counselor this might be a frequent topic of discussion. She didn't want to give up her values or lay them off to the side while working with people. She didn't want to impose them either. Her personal ethics were naturally influencing her professional/ethical identity.

Another example was where professional ethics influenced a change in the personal. In class, a student shared his recent conversation with family members about his work with some students on campus. He kept his comments to his family at a vague level. His understanding and sensitivity to confidentiality had been heightened due to the recent and ongoing conversations about confidentiality in the ethics class. As a family member pressed for more detail about his work, he stood his ground, letting his family member know that, although he recognized the importance of open communication with them, which continued to be his value, he also had begun to incorporate an aspect of his professional self—he had recognized his ethical obligation to honor the privacy of those he served on campus. From this experience he began to think more about how conversations with family members about other family members may need to change to honor his values of confidentiality and privacy.

Our professional/ethical identities evolve over time, but no matter where we are, we can improve our understanding and exploration of the core elements of our identities. The benefits of having a well-thought-out and well-articulated professional/ethical identity include providing better psychotherapy and counseling to clients, preventing burnout, and experiencing a more fulfilling and productive career.

Ethical Acculturation

We and our students have found it useful to think of our profession—our mansion—as a new culture to which we need to adapt. The culture of psychotherapy, like any culture, has its own values, customs, language, traditions, rules for appropriate and inappropriate behaviors, and ways to express gratitude, respect, and reverence. When we live and move around in our mansion, the culture of psychotherapy, our ordinary moral sense will take us only so far (Kitchener & Anderson, 2011). As we engage in the process of ethical acculturation, we are actively creating, tweaking, and expressing our professional identity.

Our adaptation to the culture of psychotherapy, which we call *ethical acculturation* (Handelsman et al., 2005), involves awareness of all the rooms and furnishings in the mansion—the personal and the professional—and the staircase of ethics. What is your sense of right and wrong professional behavior? Who have you been throughout your life, in the many types of relationships of which you have been a part? How do you integrate the ethical traditions, values, rules—in short, the culture of psychotherapy—with your own moral intuitions, values, and backgrounds?

These tasks—professional/ethical identity development and ethical accultura-tion—might take you by surprise or seem unnecessary. You might be thinking that you already have enough of a personal foundation or moral compass to be an eth-ical practitioner. For example, (a) you are very motivated to listen and to help peo-ple, (b) others tell you that you are a nice person, and (c) you have never been convicted of a felony. These statements may all be true; however, there are two major reasons why we need to engage in these tasks intentionally and mindfully. First, psychotherapy is a complex profession—the therapeutic relationship includes a unique combination of roles and behaviors. It can also include different contexts and stakeholders. Second, human beings are prone to imperfect cognitive and emo-tional processing—we often find it hard to (a) identify the ethical components of a professional decision, (b) judge accurately what a right ethical action is, and/or (c) implement our ethical judgments, especially under stressful conditions.

Practicing Ethics in the Real World: Tripping Points and Balancing Acts

In our dialogues throughout this book, we will pay attention to practicing ethics in the real world, not just studying theory or platitudes. If ethical decisions were that easy, we wouldn't need courses, books, consultants, regulatory agencies, licenses, hearings, malpractice courts, and so forth. But our professional mansion is big, complex, and constantly under renovation. Thus, ethical judgments and actions are difficult at best—and there are conditions in the real world that add to the difficulty.

The spiral staircase of ethics is sometimes treacherous, in part because human beings are not naturally good at making choices and decisions. We are prone to imperfect cognitions (think: uneven stairs), especially under conditions of uncertainty (Kahneman & Tversky, 1973)—which includes the practice of psychotherapy. We are also imperfect when emotions are involved—which they always are! Thus, our tendencies toward imperfect cognitions are magnified by emotional involvements (like slippery stairs) that include conflicts of interest, liking or disliking (of colleagues, clients, the "system," our lives, etc.), and other emotional biases. As if that weren't enough, situational factors can act like turning off the lights on the staircase—they make our climb more difficult, and they exacerbate our cognitive and emotional tendencies. We can be blind to our own blind spots.

With apologies to Gladwell (2000), we call these factors *tripping points*. They can make it hard to develop and maintain a professional identity, stay positive, make good ethical decisions in the moment, and choose good acculturation strategies.

Cultural Tripping Points

No matter what cultural groups we identify or have grown up with, we are often constrained by a limited worldview (Sue et al., 2019). Part of our exploration will be looking at the cultural filters that human beings naturally use that distort, devalue, or deny experiences of people (colleagues, clients, etc.) who are different from us in important ways. Psychotherapy itself includes values and traditions that may make more sense in some cultures. For example, many Western psychotherapeutic approaches value individuality and independence. Other worldviews value interdependence and seeking the best for the community. We aren't saying that one is better over the other. We are saying that our cultural lenses, and we all have at least one, filter our ways of seeing and understanding our clients, their world, and their experience of the world.

Stress and Tripping Points

Our human tendencies to think and act in non-rational ways are magnified under conditions of stress. When we experience situational stressors—financial pressures, peer pressure, personal relationship difficulties, illnesses, etc.—the research shows that we tend to make riskier choices (Kahneman, 2011). Thus, for example, it might be easy to know that we should maintain confidentiality, but more difficult to make that choice when we're facing uncertain promotions, tenure decisions, raises, loss of income, entreaties from families, and so forth.

Balancing Acts—Personal and Professional

Our students tell us that becoming a psychotherapist is very enjoyable and rewarding. However, they also tell us of the numerous balancing acts and frustrations in the endeavor. Each of these balancing acts has important implications for our ethical behavior.

When we become a professional, or simply start the process, many of our close relationships change. For example, your friends might expect to get expert knowledge from you and you just want to be their friend like before! However, you now have some new knowledge and you know it could be beneficial. You might even be wondering about your language. You may begin to see that you use more open-ended questions in conversations. Maybe you use more eye contact and share what you hear in a reflective manner. At some point, you might start to think, "Am I moving from giving advice, as any friend would, to giving professional opinions? Am I being a friend or a counselor when I ask a question like that? Should I even be using reflection of feeling with my friends? It seems like such a powerful tool."

Another sense in which the personal and professional need to be balanced is within our therapy relationships. Our students say things like, "You tell me to use my personality as part of treatment and yet you also say to be professional in the relationship and not just go by my personal experience." Indeed, helping people is much more than common sense or relying on your own experience. At the same time, without understanding your own tendencies, habits, and perceptions—and using your personality—psychotherapy becomes merely a mechanical process in which you risk displaying too much neutrality and objectivity and not enough compassion and genuineness. We think it is ethical to be you in the session but with a professional sense of self at the fore. Easier said than done!

The notion of technical knowledge and skill leads us to another balancing act: between humility and competence. Psychotherapists need to know an amazing amount of information about human behavior and to develop many skills to apply that knowledge. At the same time, psychotherapists need to know that they cannot help everybody and they will never know everything. Thus, they need to cultivate the virtue of humility and appreciate the limits of their competence—which is determined by their levels of knowledge and skills. However, the extremes of this balance—feeling like you know everything or feeling like you know nothing—can lead to poor practice, burnout, and ethical infractions.

As a student or practitioner exploring ethical issues, you will face yet another balancing act: between being certain and embracing ambiguity. As you initially study the ethics codes of your discipline, you will find that the codes often read like a long list of "don'ts" that should be followed blindly. Upon closer inspection, however, you will find that most of the rules are not that definite, or they contradict each other. They are often difficult to implement in simple ways. It seems like there is always "it depends" as part of the final answer. How are we supposed to behave ethically when the rules are neither clear nor absolute, or when ethical principles conflict? Answering this question takes careful study, long practice, and an open mind. We urge you to become familiar with the ethics codes of your profession, and perhaps of a few related professions. You can find links to over 100 codes or sets of guidelines at kspope.com/ethcodes/index.php. We also encourage you to draw upon your humility and seek consultation. Professionals not directly involved in a situation can often see things—like tripping points—with greater clarity. They can also be a source of accountability.

Another balance that has important ethical implications is between responsibility and respect. "They tell me I am responsible for how therapy goes," new therapists might say, "and yet they tell me that the client is in control." As psychotherapists, we must be responsible for the methods we use to help our clients, but we must also recognize that clients retain the ultimate responsibility for their own lives. Not appreciating this fact might lead us to blur the boundaries of the psychotherapeutic relationship as we take too much responsibility for clients' lives, push clients into unwise or premature choices, or impose our own values. At the same time, the spheres of responsibility are not always that clearly defined. Many of the ethical issues we explore later in the book will revolve around this issue.

Boundaries are one of the most important balancing acts that we as therapists need to master. There is a complex tension between the intimacy involved in psychotherapy and the boundaries of that intimacy. Put another way: The emotional intimacy involved in therapy exists in a very restricted range. For example, clients disclose many personal details in the relationship, but therapists typically do not. Another quality of therapeutic intimacy is that it should never be transformed into a romantic or sexual relationship, a business relationship, or even a close friendship. Respecting the boundaries of the therapy relationship is a key to effective practice (we talk more about this in Chapter 5). This balancing act is one of the most important to monitor and about which to be open to seeking supervision or consultation. It can be one of the parts of the staircase that needs additional support.

A final balancing act is between personal autonomy and professional obligations. Put simply: When are you not a psychotherapist? Are you ever off the clock? You are always a psychotherapist because it is part of you now—you live in the mansion! You are off the clock when your therapy day is done; however, your role (and the perception of some others) as a psychotherapist is still part of you. Even with our personal autonomy, we have an obligation to uphold professional responsibilities and commitments—both on and off the clock. As an analogy, think of a marriage. As a married person, when we are out with friends doing friend things, we are still married—still have obligations to that role even when our spouse is absent and we're not doing things specifically for them.

With all this conversation about tripping points, balancing acts, and developing a professional ethical identity, you might be tempted to throw up your hands and say one of these two statements: "I didn't sign up for a big mansion and climbing a spiral staircase and all that comes with it. I just want to help people." Or, "Ok, this is all interesting but I don't have the slightest clue how to explore and articulate this core of my identity, adapt to this new professional culture, or think about, let alone maneuver ethically through, all of these real-world issues and balancing acts in psychotherapy." In either scenario, you may be tempted to start walking back down the staircase. If these thoughts ring true for you, take a deep breath and let it out slowly. Relax a little and let yourself gather the strength for the next steps. We are with you on this journey and our next topic, self-care, is important to discuss.

Self-Care: The Basics

Clearly there are immense rewards for being a therapist and many find it a truly noble way to make a living. At the same time, psychotherapy is taxing and emotionally draining; authors have used phrases like "significantly stressful" (Cottone & Tarvydas, 2007, p. 123) and "inherently stressful" (Welfel, 2006, p. 58). We work with people who are unhappy, ineffective, dissatisfied, angry, anxious, and/or lonely, and who sometimes really want to stay unhappy, ineffective, dissatisfied, angry, anxious, and lonely. Under these conditions, they challenge us to be that person in their lives who brings hope, a point of connection, stability, and caring confrontation. The increments of change we may see during the therapy process are often very small. In addition, we rarely know of the positive outcomes for clients that happen long after termination. Thus, we often do not fully collect on the promise of good feelings after a job well done.

These conditions and other factors that may be out of our control (e.g., reimbursement from insurance carriers) constitute a recipe for emotional exhaustion. We need self-care strategies to prevent the harmful effects of these stresses and to help ourselves when we start to feel detached, overwhelmed, and burned out (Jevne & Williams, 1998). We need to be on guard for the telltale signs of such stress, like fleeting hopes that our clients call to cancel their appointments, impatience with our clients, and musing between sessions about going back to school to study geology or taxidermy. You need to be your own best friend and make a strong commitment to take care of yourself. Those who need your help—your clients—won't be asking you if you are getting good rest at night, taking periodic vacations, exercising regularly, or are involved in healthy personal relationships. You need to be checking in on yourself and seeking assistance from colleagues. Ask yourself questions such as these: How do you know when you are stressed? What are your telltale signs? What are your first reactions when you feel stressed? What are some ways you try to cope with stress? Would you characterize these as healthy, unhealthy, or ineffectual? What might you do differently to cope better with stress?

Myers et al. (2000) describe the concept of wellness as "a way of life oriented toward optimal health and wellbeing in which body, mind and spirit are integrated by the individual to live more fully within the human and natural community" (p. 252). Personal wellness is critical for our own wellbeing so we can draw from our core and pursue professional excellence. Spending time and effort on ourselves is part of our ethical obligation, in addition to the time and effort we spend on behalf of our clients. As Skovholt and Trotter-Mathison (2016) state, "Maintaining oneself personally is necessary to function effectively in a professional role. By itself, this idea can help those in the caring fields feel less selfish when meeting the needs of the self" (p. 161). In an important sense, wellness and self-care are to stress reduction as positive ethics is to ethics—it allows us to go beyond the minimum and reach a higher level.

As a way to evaluate your self-care, consider the following list of categories. For each category, give yourself a rating of 0–5, with 0 meaning "no self-care" and 5 meaning "good self-care" in the category.

_____ I encourage myself to experience emotions—all kinds of emotions.
_____ I have my finances in good to great shape.
_____ I laugh at least once during each day.
_____ I give other people, as well as myself, a compliment most every day.
_____ I have a healthy diet when it comes to food.
_____ I walk and/or get exercise sometime during my day.
_____ I hydrate regularly with water.
_____ I get sufficient sleep on a regular basis.
_____ I have hobbies or activities that I do only for fun.
_____ I keep my life's priorities front and center and don't let the tyranny of the urgent draw me off course.
_____ I stop and just breathe when my day starts to feel stressful.
_____ I give myself permission to be alone when I need solitary time.
_____ I turn my phone off.
_____ I take time to foster my spiritual or religious self.
_____ I have at least one healthy relationship in my life.

Now go back over your list and see if there are any scores you wish to change. If yes, write an action plan for one of those items. Keep this list handy so that you can retrieve it on a regular basis. We would suggest that you do this activity at least twice a year.

In spite of the inherent stress of psychotherapy, there are ways to stay vibrant in the profession. Skovholt and Trotter-Mathison (2016) encourage professionals to seek out those experiences in their personal lives that promote happiness, fervor, energy, and tranquility. Of course, the list you develop to experience these will likely look different from your colleagues' or classmates'. That's fine. The key is to make the list and then implement your list on a regular basis. It is also important to remember that your list will change over the years as you develop as a person and a professional. And remember to have lots of items on your list that are not connected to your professional activities! Your list should be a personal one, not a professional one.

How to Get the Most Out of This Book

We have written this book to be different from other ethics books, some of which you may be using along with this one. The first difference is that this book is not discipline-specific. We have written it for all who are or will be performing psychotherapy, including counselors, marriage and family therapists, psychiatrists, psychologists, social workers, and others. Thus, we will not provide as comprehensive a guide to discipline-specific ethical situations.

The second difference is that this book is not a set of rules to follow in every situation. We will provide some answers about what to do in some situations, but we are more interested in helping you develop your ability to (a) recognize ethical issues because you are more sensitized to them, (b) think about ethical issues from a knowledgeable position, (c) integrate what you read in the ethics codes with who you are as a person and professional, and (d) develop the character strengths to act in concert with your convictions. To the extent that we achieve these goals, you will be more likely to follow your ethics codes now and as they evolve in the future.

Third, we wrote this book with you in mind. We want to help you accurately know yourself, successfully acculturate to the world of psychotherapy, and be prepared to actualize your ethical ideals in practice. You can think of this approach with three A's: activity, awareness, and aspiration.

Activity

We don't know you. We don't know the courses you have taken or the disciplines you have studied. Regardless, we want to help you uncover, explore, and articulate what is in your core and consider how to integrate your ethical and professional selves in some systematic, integrative, and fulfilling ways. Although we focus on universal ethical issues that all psychotherapists face, your professional/ethical identity is yours alone. We invite you to be partners with us and to explore your identity actively. Indeed, the key to your learning experience will be your reactions to what we have written. To this end, we have provided three types of activities throughout the book.

The first activity is titled *Journal Entries*. This activity offers the most formal way to explore and take more responsibility for your learning from this book. You can keep your journal in a hard-copy notebook, a computer file, or on Instagram. The format doesn't matter—what matters is taking the opportunities to self-reflect and explore. We will make some suggestions for journal entries, but we encourage you to be willing to write down some of your reactions and thoughts about what you read. Some of you might do this already in various aspects of your life. Or, you may never have tried writing stuff down. You might feel more comfortable talking through your thoughts. You may want to record your thoughts via voice and transcribe them later. The point is, we think it's important for you to reflect, to think more intentionally, mindfully, and deeply about the issues we're exploring. We encourage you to avoid the human tendency to read a passage and immediately say things like, "Got it," or "Yep, that's me!"

The second type of activity we call *Food for Thought*. These are opportunities for you to sit back and reflect upon what you're reading and how you relate to it. Although not as formal as journal entries, these reflections can really contribute to your learning. You might think of them as extra consideration of the next step on the staircase, whereas the journal entries involve building handrails or sanding down rough edges on the steps.

The third type of activity we call *Red Flag* and *Green Flag* stories, which we introduce in Chapter 4. This is where we articulate some of the tripping points (red flags) and ways to prevent, mitigate, or transcend tripping points and achieve ethical excellence (green flags). The flag stories contain specific examples of behaviors and attitudes that you can think about, react to, and expand upon.

If you are reading this book for a class, your professor may ask you to do some additional entries or exercises, or ask you to share your work as part of a class discussion. The purpose of every activity is to facilitate the development of your professional/ethical identity and ethical acculturation—to explore yourself, the culture of psychotherapy, and/or the relationship between the two. As you respond to our prompts, remember that there are very few clearly right or wrong answers; we've left most of the questions open-ended to facilitate your exploration.

A note about the process of activities: We encourage you to take your time and reflect on what is being asked or what we offer through one of the flag stories. You don't want to feel like it is absolutely necessary to answer every question in every activity or even to do every activity. You choose what is most meaningful at this time, knowing that you may come back to the chapter at a later time to do some additional reflection. However, we believe the more you do, the more you will benefit from this book. Think of these activities as walking up some stairs on the staircase or entering and exploring one of the rooms in the mansion. We intend the exercises to have multiple benefits, including growing self-understanding about who you are and who you want to be as an ethical professional.

Awareness

We ask you to keep an open mind and to continue expanding your awareness. For example, in our activities we sometimes ask you to take different perspectives. We ask you to respond as a therapist, but we will also ask you to put yourself in different positions or roles like that of a client, a colleague, a member of an ethics committee, a member of the public, and so forth. These perspectives will help you understand the complexity and uniqueness of psychotherapy and build your ethical sensitivity. Another example: We ask you to be aware of your potential tripping points—realizing that all human beings have them.

Most of our suggestions will be worded in such a way as to apply primarily to beginning therapists. However, we think practicing psychotherapists would do well to revisit this book on a regular basis. If you are an experienced therapist you can easily adapt the activities by thinking about the next stage of your career as a renewal or re-entry into a changing professional culture. But do not modify the activities too much! There is much to be gained from moving back a few steps and casting fresh eyes upon steps that we believe we have already covered.

Aspiration

In spite of the difficulties inherent in navigating your new mansion, we hope you see developing your ethical identity as a positive and personal venture rather than an alienating attempt to follow a disembodied set of rules (Handelsman et al., 2009). For example, it is important for psychotherapists to include the informed consent process in the first session and it is an unethical choice not to do so. However, sometimes new psychotherapists skip the informed consent process because they aren't comfortable with talking about confidentiality and its limits. Other therapists skip it because they believe it detracts from building the relationship with clients. Although we understand these concerns, a more positive and aspirational perspective is honoring the client and their right to be truly informed and addressing the difficult questions that might come with limits to confidentiality. Avoidance of confidentiality issues and upfront conversations about the limits work against our desire to produce beneficial therapeutic outcomes and to act in clients' best interests. Clients need to know what is promised and what is not promised in the therapy relationship.

Journal Entry: *Chapter Reflections*

Here is your first journal entry. We have posed some questions to help you reflect on this chapter:

- How did you react to this first chapter?
- What surprised you about what we said?

- What parts of the chapter/discussion seemed to make the most sense and what parts were counterintuitive?
- Did you find yourself getting defensive at anything we said? If yes, what?
- What are you most looking forward to about this book: the mansion and its rooms, the spiral staircase? What are you least looking forward to?

This is a journal entry that you can repeat at the end of *every* chapter!

Food for Thought: *Big Questions*

Right now, take a few minutes and reflect on these big questions, which we will return to at various points in the book:

- What do you see as important when it comes to ethics?
- What do you think of when you think of "professional ethics"?
- What you think professional ethics includes?
- What is the relationship, as you think of it, between your personal morality and your professional ethics?
- How do you see yourself in relationship to professional ethics?
- What part does ethics play in your current and future professional identity?
- What might be your ethical weak spots in your profession? What kind of mistakes might you make?
- When are you—or might you be—not at your best when making ethical decisions? What happens at those times?

Coming Attractions

In Chapters 1 and 2 we ask you to think more about you and your background and how it might prepare you for your professional roles. In Chapter 3 we will discuss in more detail the process of acculturation and how to develop your professional identity. Readers who want a broad overview before getting into specifics may want to read Chapter 3 first.

Part I
Taking Stock

1

Basics of Awareness
Knowing Yourself and Your Core

Our dialogue with you in this chapter is about *you*. What have you noticed about *you* in the community comprising the mansion? What do you notice about *you* in the elegant mansion itself? What have you noticed about *your* curiosity regarding the many rooms? And what have you noticed about *you* and *your* climb up the spiral staircase thus far?

Our own ethics students are often surprised when they begin our courses by exploring (by writing and discussing) the question, "Who are you?" Some students initially respond with some variation of, "Well, I'm a student, a partner, a parent, a server at a restaurant, a retired service person." These responses are about roles in life. They are important aspects of identity; however, they aren't really about the students at their *core*. Then we push a little harder: "Who are you really?" Students begin to describe aspects of their character. For example, "I'm a nice person," or I'm a curious person," or "I'm a fixer." Now we're moving! Another little push: "What motivates you? What values do you hold that prompt you to be a nice person, a curious person, a fixer?" Now students are exploring the core of who they are: their *identity*.

Professional Identity and the Moral Core

Burke (2003) describes identity as "what it means to be who one is" (p. 1). Blasi (1984) suggests that identity is "rooted in the core of one's being" and is an "organization of self-related information" (p. 130). According to Blasi, the organized, self-related data are so critical that without them "the individual would see himself or herself to be radically different; those so central that one could not even imagine being deprived of them; those whose loss would be considered and felt as irreparable" (p. 131).

Part of our identity is our moral core—our notions of right and wrong. Blasi (1984) suggests that moral/ethical ideals "are powerless if they are not rooted in a moral self" (p. 130). He also suggests one's moral identity fuels (or is the moral/ethical motivation for) one's moral/ethical action. To move from "powerless" to powerful or ethically excellent, we start with exploring and discovering your core—your essential moral self.

In our experience, the opportunity to uncover, explore, and articulate what resides in their core makes our students more able to think about how they fit with the profession, what it means to be part of the profession, and, consequently, how best to serve their clients, patients, students, consultees, and the broader society. We understand that you might be anxious to skip this part of your experience on the staircase—"Let's just get to the good stuff!"—but these steps provide a critical root for growing your professional/ethical identity.

Developing a professional/ethical identity takes effort. We've discovered students typically fall into one of the following groups: Some students have never really considered some of the deeper levels of their identities. If they have done some good thinking, they haven't really articulated their thoughts. Others can articulate what's there, but they haven't stopped to assess what is fundamental, missing, or problematic in their core. The last group includes those who haven't explored the relationship between their core (central, non-negotiable) identity and its relationship to their developing professional identity.

Your awareness of your core, moral self provides the foundation for your professional identity—including your motivations, needs, values, and social identities. Knowledge of your core self helps you traverse the spiral staircase—to think about your relationship to the profession, to sustain your professional ethical identity for the long term, and to practice positive ethics. Thus, the foundation of a healthy and solid professional identity begins with understanding what's in your core. Let's start, or continue, your exploration with some reflecting.

Food for Thought: *Who Are You?*

Take a few minutes to reflect on some of the following questions:

- Who are you really?
- What does it mean to be you?
- What are some of your ethics and morals of origin (from your family) that continue to influence how you see the world?
- Think about your last big decision. What needs and motivations influenced your thinking and your final choice?

Needs and Motivations

Your motivations for being a psychotherapist, and the needs that drive your motivations, are analogous to the fuel or energy that prompts you to enter the mansion and climb the spiral staircase. These needs and motivations are many and varied, including what Murray (1938) called *secondary needs*, such as the need for achievement, gaining and/or retaining materials, power or autonomy, affection-giving and receiving, nurturance, gaining knowledge and sharing it with others. These needs generate motivations for various professional activities, including gaining knowledge and helping others grow.

When we review statements of interest from prospective graduate students, we frequently come across a number of honorable motivations. These noble motivations usually match up well with the personal needs and stated experiences of students: "I like to help people and seem to be pretty good at it. My friends tell me I am a natural. I think this makes me a good match for being a therapist," or, "My friends typically look to me for guidance. If they have a problem, I'm the one they contact."

Other needs and motives do not appear on graduate school applications, because they don't seem relevant or because students are a little ashamed of them. For example, most people want (and need!) to earn money to make a living. A need for achievement might motivate people to enter a profession that enjoys some prestige.

Some of our needs and motives can remain hidden, even from us. We might have an unconscious need to be in power; doing therapy is a way to exert our power in other people's lives.

It is worth the time to uncover the personal needs that drive our professional ambitions (Bashe et al., 2007). Here's an example of why it's important to understand personal needs. This is from Sharon:

> I realized during my internship year that one of my motivations to become a psychotherapist grew out of a subconscious drive to make sense of my own family dynamics. This realization came to light while working with an estranged couple. I saw the husband as non-emotional and aloof, and the wife as emotionally needy, neglected, and fragile. I felt good about my work with this couple until my supervisor reviewed the latest session. At one point, she stopped the recording and pointed out how I had really aligned myself with the wife and joined her in blaming her husband for their marriage problems. My first response was shock. My next response was "Ouch!" My professional ego had been pinched! My subconscious need to "fix" a family-of-origin relationship compromised my ability to connect with the husband of this couple. I wasn't listening well and I was not being helpful to my clients. In this case, my purely personal need to make sense of my parents' relationship inhibited my professional motivation to do good work.

Some personal needs and motivations are appropriate—in the right amount—and drive helpful professional behavior. For an analogy, think of nitroglycerine: In small doses, it can keep people alive. In larger doses, it's deadly. Small doses of some personal needs, balanced with professional motivations and sensitivity, will work well. For example, a little psychological voyeurism (wanting to hear about other people's private lives) might be a good thing when combined with compassion, respect, humility, helping, and objectivity. The voyeurism might help you develop respect. It might keep you interested. Another example is your financial and power needs. These two needs, used appropriately, allow you to do what you do and to achieve your larger goals of helping and service.

The bottom line: Psychotherapy is a profession, which means you don't just get to do what you want to do. Although your personal needs play a role, your primary motivations need to be professional and moral (Kitchener & Anderson, 2011; Rest, 1983, 1984, 1994).

Journal Entry: *Needs and Motivations*

We now ask you to dig deep and explore some of the most personal elements of your core. Therefore, we suggest that you complete at least the first two parts of this entry in a quiet, private place where you can be honest with yourself.

Part 1:   What personal needs might you be meeting by being or becoming a psychotherapist? When you think back to completing your application for graduate school, what were your top three motivations for applying—for wanting to be a therapist? Are these motivations still present? Since applying to graduate school, what other needs and motivations have become apparent to you that surprise you? What needs and motivations *may* you have that you haven't thought of?

Be inclusive in your list of needs and motivations. You may want to revisit the list of secondary needs above as you make your list. When you list your motivations, include the noble ones you discussed on your application. Then, let your guard down to include the less noble needs and resulting motivations. For example, you may like the idea of (a) a nice office rather than a cubicle, (b) prestige and status, (c) being needed, (d) hearing other people's stories, (e) demonstrating expertise or power in a relationship, and/or (f) saving others from the kind of family you had. Go beyond what you know—speculate about some needs and motivations that you might have even if you are not in touch with them at the moment. Remember Sharon's story? If she had done this exercise during her training before internship, she might have uncovered the hidden need to understand family dynamics and been less likely to align herself with only one person of the couple.

Part 2:   With your list of needs and motivations in front of you, think about how important each one is or might be. Rate each need and motivation on a scale from 1 to 5, with one being "just a little important," and 5 being "absolutely critical to my being a therapist." One way to make these judgments is to ask yourself how you would feel about being a therapist if a particular need or motivation were not satisfied. For example, if "having a big office with nice furniture" is on your list, what would it do to your desire to be a therapist if we told you (just for the sake of argument) that that motivation would definitely not be satisfied during your career?

Values

Like needs and motivations, values can range from noble to base. Schwartz (1994) identified 10 groupings of values:

- Power (authority, wealth, social recognition)
- Achievement (ambition, competence, success)
- Hedonsim (pursuit of pleasure, enjoyment, gratification of desires)
- Stimulation (variety, excitement, novelty)
- Self-direction (creativity, independence, self-respect)
- Universalism (social justice, equality, wisdom, environmental concern)
- Benevolence (honesty, helpfulness, loyalty)
- Conformity (politeness, obedience, self-discipline/restraint)
- Tradition (respect for tradition and the status quo, acceptance of customs)
- Security (safety, stability of society).

We can understand values in two ways: values as preferences and values as principles (Parks & Guay, 2009). Values as preferences are personal choices about desirability. They are subjective and can easily change over time. Values as principles are more objective and consistent. We can call them moral values, and they are guides to how people ought to behave (Parks & Guay, 2009, p. 676). Moral values have to do with your relationships to other people: helping them, respecting them, and fulfilling duties.

Some of your moral values are personal and learned from your family of origin, your religious traditions, and other sources. Some of your values are, or will be, purely professional—learned from the socialization process within professional contexts. Some of your values will overlap and be a combination of personal and professional values.

Probably some of your values revolve around the human condition and the desire to see people thrive and grow. Obviously, these values match well with many of the goals of psychotherapy—they also drive, in part, your motivation to be a therapist. Some of your values, however, revolve around financial, social, and personal success and stability. Being a successful psychotherapist is clearly a way to actualize these values. The bottom line is that our values are complex; thus, the likelihood of dealing with conflicting values is high. Indeed, one way to assess and better understand our values is to explore the choices we make when values conflict with other values and/or motives (Abeles, 1980). For example, you might believe that having nice things is a good thing and you value having a nice office in which to work, but your value and motivation to help people without access to mental health care keep you working at the local mental health center for a lower salary than you could earn in private practice.

Journal Entry: *Values and Values Conflicts*

Similar to the list of needs and motivations you considered around being a therapist, generate a list of your values—both personal and professional. You might use the list identified by Schwartz. After you've created your list, rank them based on their importance. Which ones are personally most important? Which ones are personally least important? Now, narrow your focus to professional values: When you think about fulfilling the role of therapist, which values are most important? Make note of the overlap and potential conflicts between (and within!) your lists of personal and professional values.

These lists of needs, motivations and values are part of your core—the foundation of your professional/ethical identity. A good understanding of your core helps you shoot for the ethical ideal (not perfection, by the way)—setting your goals, understanding the tripping points along the way, and choosing excellent behaviors.

However, not all of your needs, motivations, and values as a professional are satisfied at any given time. For example, your value of helping, your motivation of wanting to see them grow, and your need to feel successful will not be fully actualized when you don't see clients improving, or improving as quickly as you think they could. Staying mindful of your full set of needs, motivations, and values may help ground you during these times of discouragement.

It is important to know the difference between having values and the expression or implementation of those values. Sometimes it will appear that the values you hold conflict with those of the psychotherapy profession. However, the issue may be one of expression rather than the values themselves. For example: We may value compassion, but we cannot show our compassion with clients in the same way we do with friends (hugging, lending money, sharing our problems, etc.). Many of the situations and issues we explore throughout the book, about boundaries, confidentiality, and so forth, will involve how we express our values differently in professional contexts. Many will also involve actual conflicts of values.

Food for Thought: *Exploring Personal Needs, Motivations, and Values*

A client of yours is working on some anxiety about her local acting job. The client tells you wonderful, funny stories about her life and family. You are fascinated, at times spellbound, by the client's dramatic way of speaking. She is a pleasure to work with because she is professionally rewarding—she's making progress in therapy—and personally engaging. Several months later, the client appears on a local news program telling those same stories as part of her one-person show. Within a few months, your now-former client has made it big! You see her now on national talk shows; she even refers to her "shrink" in some of her interviews. You can't help but feel the urge (as any human being would) to brag to your friends that you're the "shrink" and that you helped her work through her anxiety to get to where she is today.

   Explore your needs, motivations, and values: Why do you want to tell others? What need might telling others meet? To feel powerful, important? To impress your friends? To become, perhaps, a bit of a celebrity yourself? What values come to mind as you explore the urge to share this little bit of information? Keep exploring and speculating until you gain some new insights into your needs, motivations, and values. What *might* be there? What are the new insights and how do/might they influence your understanding of your core and your professional/ethical identity?

Virtues

We hope your exploration so far—these first stairs and first rooms of your mansion—has been an insightful experience. You know more about yourself now and that probably feels good, if somewhat daunting. Now, let's take the next steps and explore your core in terms of personal traits, characteristics, or habits—in other words, your *virtues*. Philosophers, ethicists, and psychologists from at least the time of Aristotle have identified important virtues (Jordan & Meara, 1990; Meara et al., 1996; Peterson & Seligman, 2004; Vasquez, 1996), many of which are relevant and desirable for psychotherapists.

   Peterson and Seligman (2004) have outlined six basic virtues along with associated character strengths, outlined in Table 1.1. For our purposes, we can consider all of them virtues. This is not an exhaustive list, and we invite you to think of others that might be important for you.

Table 1.1 Virtues and Character Strengths (From Peterson & Seligman, 2004).

I. Wisdom and knowledge
   A. Creativity
   B. Curiosity
   C. Open-mindedness
   D. Love of learning
   E. Perspective
II. Courage
   A. Bravery
   B. Persistence
   C. Integrity
   D. Vitality
III. Humanity
   A. Love
   B. Kindness
   C. Social intelligence
IV. Justice
   A. Citizenship
   B. Fairness
   C. Leadership
V. Temperance
   A. Forgiveness
   B. Humility
   C. Prudence
   D. Self-regulation
VI. Transcendence
   A. Appreciation of beauty and excellence
   B. Gratitude
   C. Hope
   D. Humor
   E. Spirituality

As you consider your (current and future) virtues and their relationship to your professional behavior, keep a few important points in mind. First, others can only infer our virtues from our behavior. We may not be good at expressing our virtues, or the right combination of virtues in the right amounts. Thus, we may think we are acting in accordance with our highest virtues, but others—colleagues, clients, state licensing boards—might perceive a failure of virtue. In these situations, our *intent* to display virtues is not as important as the behavior itself. For example, we may display courage in the wrong way by lying in court to secure our client's custody of their children. "I was trying to be helpful" is not usually a good defense of unethical actions. When choosing actions, we need to consider the virtues that it *looks like* we're expressing, not only the ones that we are intending to express.

Second, too much or too little of a virtue can be problematic. For example, too little compassion leads to indifference and too much compassion may lead to problems like taking too much responsibility for clients or enabling their self-defeating behaviors. Another example: Too little humility leads to arrogance and too much humility can lead to self-debasement and timidity.

Third, virtues do not exist in isolation; most behaviors reflect multiple virtues in combination. Consider the virtue of truthfulness. Sometimes we don't tell a client the entire truth. For instance, we may not tell a client in couples therapy what their partner said about them in a private therapy session. Our virtue of truthfulness is tempered by virtues such as respectfulness (the partner shared impressions in private and expects their privacy to be respected) and prudence (sharing the information at this time in therapy may cause more harm than good). The ability to consider and express the right combinations and amounts of virtues is a virtue in itself—called *practical wisdom.*

We suggest that, along with practical wisdom, the virtues of courage (Angelou, cited in Ju, 2008), integrity, humility, and prudence are central. Courage is necessary for us to be in contact with our core, even in difficult situations, and to exercise our practical wisdom consistently. Integrity is the state of having our other virtues in proper proportions and balance. Humility is the awareness that we may not be fully competent, aware, and virtuous in every situation. Prudence refers to the habit of acting cautiously, with due regard to the potential consequences of our behavior. Some other virtues that psychotherapists might cultivate include compassion, respectfulness, and truthfulness.

Journal Entry: *Virtues*

As we did with needs, motives, and values, we can separate virtues into personal and professional, with a subset of moral virtues. We invite you to consider the moral virtues that are currently part of your core and those you wish to cultivate in your professional activities.

Part 1: Write down the list of virtues from Table 1.1, along with any others you want to consider. Next to each one of them, rank how well you express that virtue in your life—which includes having the right amount of the virtue, and in optimal combination with other virtues. (You might want to rank them in terms of how much *others* would say you express these virtues.) The scale runs from 1 to 10 (1—not at all to 10—expressed every possible time). For those virtues you demonstrate frequently, answer this question: "When I don't express _____ as a virtue, I end up being and/or feeling _____." For example, if you consider yourself a compassionate person most of the time, when you are not compassionate you might feel (a) frustrated and get in a person's way by making a decision for them or (b) apathetic and decide to distance yourself and not provide support or guidance they might need.

Part 2:   Think about several kinds of situations you face in your life and see if there are variations in your expression of virtues. For example, if you thought of truthfulness, how does the amount or expression of truthfulness change depending upon the people you are dealing with, the type of situation, the kinds of behavior called for, and other considerations? Think, for example, about somebody you are very close to, somebody with whom you have a professional relationship, and somebody who is merely an acquaintance. Think about a work situation, a personal situation, and/or a family situation.

Part 3:
- What would your friends consider your greatest virtue? Your weakest?
- What do you hope your clients will say about your virtues?
- What do you hope your colleagues will say about your virtues?
- What virtues will you most want to develop in your role as a psychotherapist?
- What is your plan for how you might develop these virtues?

Social Identities

Social identities refer to the sense of who we are, based on group membership, and are central aspects of identity for many of us. The following is a short list of social identities: race, ethnicity, gender, social class, religion, worldview, able-bodiedness, and sexual orientation. Social identities could include assumptions, biases, and blind spots regarding how we view both ourselves and others. We encourage you to take some time, perhaps in your journal, to uncover and explore how these identities contribute to your core and how they will contribute to your professional/ethical identity. We will address social identities and issues of privilege and oppression in Chapter 2.

The Ethics Autobiography—Part 1

Along with our colleagues, we (Bashe et al., 2007) have used the ethics autobiography frequently over the years in our undergraduate and graduate ethics courses. We use it in our class discussions, and we invite you to use it as one way to self-reflect about your core and your ethical identity. Think of it as a walking stick as you climb the staircase!

We'll introduce Part 2 of the autobiography in Chapter 4, after we've introduced the basics of the culture of psychotherapy. For now, Part 1 is a chance to apply much of what you have explored of your needs, motivations, values, virtues, and social identities. In addition, there are some new items for you to consider.

Journal Entry: *Ethics Autobiography—Part 1*

Put the following on the top of a new page in your journal: Name, date, where you are in your professional journey (graduate school, employment, newly licensed, etc.), and anything else that will help make a connection for you about the time and place of this journal entry.

Here are some questions that form the basis of your ethics autobiography. You need not address them all, or in order. After all, it's *your* autobiography. You might want to refer to some of your previous journal entries, but feel free to go beyond them and integrate them.

1. What personal needs will be met (or are being met) by becoming (being) a psychotherapist? What is your sense of why those needs exist?
2. What motivations, values, virtues, and social identities are most important to you, as a person, in your relationships with other people?
3. What are the origins of these motivations, values, virtues, etc.? Take some time on this one. For example, how did you learn about values and develop them? How did you acquire the motivations you have for being a psychotherapist?
4. What drives your notions of right and wrong? You might draw upon a story about yourself that highlights your sense of right and wrong behavior. Tell the story—what actually happened—and describe how you thought about right and wrong. You might want to discuss how the story would have gone if a similar situation arose in a different context, and how and why you might behave differently.
5. In terms of your social identities, how similar are your needs, motivations, values, and virtues to those of other members of the cultures to which you belong? Here, you can think broadly about culture. Mitch, for example, belongs to the cultures of trumpet players, contact lens wearers, and full professors.
6. What experiences have you had with members of cultures to which you do not belong and their notions of right and wrong? What feelings did you have about those experiences and about the members of those other cultures?

7. At this stage in your professional journey, what would you consider examples of right and wrong *professional* behavior?

8. Where do your ideas of right and wrong professional behavior come from?

9. How might your motivations, values, virtues, and social identities that you wrote about in questions 1–3 influence your decisions about right and wrong professional behavior?

10. As you've answered the preceding questions, what thoughts and feelings are stirred in you? How do your journal entries about needs, motivations, and values sound now as you re-read them?

What you've written is the beginning of a rough draft of your autobiography. Your autobiography, like your growth and development as a professional, will never be finished; your experiences, thoughts, and perspectives will change over time. So keep this portion of your journal accessible, as you will have occasion to refer back to it, reconceptualize it, and revise it many times.

2

Basics of Awareness
Privilege, Discrimination, Oppression, and Social Justice

Social awareness, which includes issues of privilege, discrimination, oppression, and social justice, permeates many of the rooms in our mansion, and we need to create light around these issues to traverse the spiral staircase. Most of us have strong emotional reactions to literature, conversations, and media presentations that highlight such issues as racism, discrimination, and White supremacy. These emotions will vary depending on our social identities, socialization, experiences, and differences in worldview. Sue et al. (2019) remind us that being aware of our clients' identities and their worldviews is critical, but even more critical is being aware of our own reactions to differing worldviews and issues of privilege, racism, discrimination, and oppression.

We are here to join you. As part of that, we realize that we need to be clear about our own potential tripping points. As two White, able-bodied, middle income, educated people who have our own biases, assumptions, and other points of privilege, we realize that we might be more likely to *not* see or call out all the possible tripping points along the way; however, we are committed to address what we do know and further the dialogue with you as we climb.

Food for Thought: *Your Favorite and Not-So-Favorite Client*

Clients have different identities and descriptors (e.g., tall, short, female, male, Asian, Black, Hispanic, Native American, White, heterosexual, LGBTQ, homeless, rich, able-bodied, wheelchair user, motivated, unmotivated, clean, dirty, attractive, unattractive, old, young, genteel, foul-mouthed, thin, obese, urban, rural, liberal, conservative, communist, socialist, Christian, Jewish, Muslim, Hindu, orthodox, atheist, truck-driver, rock star, psychotherapist). Add whatever other identities and descriptors that come to mind. Picture (based on identities and descriptors) the "perfect" client from your view. List the emotions/feelings you have as you anticipate being in a session with this person. What's in your core that prompts these emotions?

Next, picture your least favorite client (again based on identities and descriptors). Once again, list all the emotions/feelings you might have as you anticipate seeing this person. What's prompted them from your core? Compare your lists of emotions and what motivated them. These emotions are a critical part of our experience with clients. If we let them, they can inform us about our prejudices, biases, preferences, and values.

Privilege

We begin this section with a story by Sharon:

> I want to share with you some of my journey of coming to see my privilege (for an extended version of this story, see Anderson, 2018), which has been a very important part of my own uncovering and exploring my core and developing my professional ethical identity. I share this story to highlight several features and tripping points of ascending my own spiral staircase: First, becoming aware of one's point(s) of privilege can be uncomfortable. Second, being willing to have what I call "difficult dialogues" with individuals different from ourselves about points of privilege, discrimination, and oppression is necessary. These dialogues help reveal values and motivations in our core. Third, growing awareness in the area of privilege, oppression, and discrimination is a journey that never ends—it is an ongoing process. Allowing our inner selves to let down the defenses and see privilege, oppression, and discrimination in a subjective way (including ourselves in the mix) is an important first step in the process. Fourth, awareness is only the beginning—action to address issues of discrimination and oppression needs to come next.
>
> Context:
>
> My family of origin is of White European descent, Christian, lower-middle class, and farmers/ranchers. I was raised in a mostly all-White, low- to middle-income, rural community. The country church I attended was all White and the K-12 school I attended was mostly White with only a handful of students and one staff member—the janitor—who identified as Mexican. My worldview was built on what I knew and had experienced as a White, Christian, heterosexual, non-disabled, lower-middle-class female.
>
> My world and experiences expanded greatly through a position with federally funded programs (e.g., Upward Bound) after obtaining my master's. I experienced disruptions of my socialization during those seven years due to the population we served and my colleagues of color. My doctoral experience brought more opportunities for disruption by way of the literature I read, friendships I forged, and a faculty member of color. However, my blindness to White privilege was deep in my core. Although I don't

recall ever hearing my parents or other adult family members make overt derogatory remarks about people of color, I also don't recall any discussions about inequality, discrimination, oppression, or privilege. My family's view on success and hard work was based on the Protestant work ethic and the "pull yourself up by your bootstraps" notion. I believed this, too.

White privilege revealed:

Two events occurred that disrupted my blindness to White privilege. The first event, during my doctoral program, planted an important seed for the second event, a defining moment that occurred some years later. Allow me to describe them:

A seed planted: A friend, who identifies as an African-American female and who worked with me in Upward Bound, called me one night and told me about a recent experience she had had at a fast-food restaurant. My friend was in the front of the line, ready to order her food. "I am standing right there ready to order and the employee, a White woman, looked right past me and asked this person who was right behind me and who just happened to be White, 'May I help you?' …. She just ignored me—like I wasn't even there." My friend was hurt and angry, and clearly believed the act was discriminatory and oppressive.

Although I heard the anger and hurt in my friend's voice, I remember having a difficult time accepting her explanation of the event. I remembered thinking (but not saying), "I'm sure you're mistaken. People aren't that rude. I'll bet the employee just thought you were still deciding on your order and wanted to keep the line moving."

Defining moment:

After completing my doctorate and spending a year in the Midwest as a staff psychologist at a university counseling center, I received a faculty appointment at Colorado State University. There I developed a friendship with a colleague who identifies as a Black female. My colleague and I would have what I call "difficult dialogues." She wanted me to hear her stories and the stories of others who are (un)seen and treated differently because of their skin color. I wanted to deflect the issues of oppression and discrimination by claiming that White people are treated poorly as well. I would argue for what I called then reverse discrimination.

One day while at lunch at a restaurant, we decided to check into the possibility of using that restaurant as a meeting place for future conversations that would include our colleagues. We started to look for an employee of the establishment. The following few seconds disrupted how I understood oppression as an intellectual concept and made it, in my eyes, a reality. A few feet in front of me, my colleague approached the receptionist, a White woman, to inquire about the cost and availability of the facility. The receptionist craned her neck to look around my colleague, as if she wasn't there, and then asked me, "How can I help you?" As this scene played out before me, so did a flashback of the conversation with my friend, some 10 years earlier, who told me about her experience of being invisible at the fast-food restaurant. For various reasons, my psychological defenses were down enough to see how my white skin made me visible *and how my colleague's black skin made her invisible. This was really a starting point for my awareness about my White privilege and a person of color's oppression.*

Peggy McIntosh, a research scientist at the Wellesley Centers for Women and a pioneer in the field, coined the term "White privilege" (1990) when she realized that as a White person she had access, opportunities, and advantages that others did not. She described White privilege as that "invisible package of unearned assets" which is like a "weightless knapsack of special provisions, maps, passports, codebooks, visas, clothes, tools, and blank checks" that those of us who have white skin "can count on cashing in each day" and to which we "remain oblivious" (p. 31).

Each one of us has our own socialization experience. Sharon's blindness to White privilege and other privilege statuses originated in her socialization process. As Harro (2013) suggests, socialization within a system of oppression is "pervasive … consistent … circular … self-perpetuating … and invisible" (p. 45). During the socialization process, Minnich states that White people are taught to see their lives "as morally neutral, normative, and average, and also ideal" (cited in McIntosh, 2000, p. 32). Although White people might not have heard their family of origin make overt derogatory remarks about people whose lives are different from theirs, the subtext might have been one of White superiority or "fear of 'the other'" (Zetzer, 2018, p. 9).

White privilege is just one point of privilege. Other points include gender privilege, able-bodied privilege, economic privilege, Christian privilege, and heterosexual privilege. Because we all have multiple identities, we may experience privilege in some areas (where we are part of a dominant group) while we experience discrimination or oppression in others (Lo, 2011). We can experience a type of "mental whiplash, alternating … between disadvantaged and privileged group memberships" (Liddle, 2011, p. 251). We might even have both experiences at the same time in the same place.

Food for Thought: *Your Own Invisible Knapsack of Privilege*

Sometimes it is uncomfortable to think of ourselves as having advantages in life or as living with unearned assets that provide us opportunities that others do not have. We'd like to give you an opportunity to explore what might be in your own "knapsack of privilege" by assessing how your experience matches the statements below. The more you respond in the affirmative, the more likely you are to have one or more points of privilege (gender privilege, able-bodied privilege, economic privilege, heterosexual privilege, religious privilege, White privilege, etc.).

- In meetings or gatherings, my ideas or comments are recognized.
- I can expect to earn my pay based on the work I do—equivalent to what my colleagues earn.
- I can go out to a place of business, a restaurant, or an event and not worry about accessibility.
- I can go to restaurant or movie and not need someone to read the menu or list of showings.
- I can plan regular trips to the grocery store without concerns of how I will pay the bill.
- I can travel, purchase items, go out for entertainment (i.e., have financial resources) without concern about how I will purchase the necessities for daily living.
- I can speak in public and not have someone ask me where I am from.
- I can hold my partner's hand in social contexts without concern.
- I can go to public places and not have people question my gender.
- I can attend the church or place of worship I desire.
- I can speak for myself as an individual and not feel like I am representing a group of people with my same skin color (or gender, religion, etc.).
- I can find plenty of literature that highlights my heritage.

Without some prompting, we might remain oblivious to our invisible knapsack of privilege. This state of unawareness may be an outcome of learning. McIntosh states it this way: "As a White person, I realized I had been taught about racism as something that puts others at a disadvantage, but had been taught not to see one of its corollary aspects, white privilege, which puts me at an advantage" (p. 31). Dr. McIntosh is not alone in this experience. In our personal contexts, we may have not learned to notice those ways we have "advantages," and may just come to see them as the expected. When we don't see our own points of privilege, we will likely find it difficult to see discrimination against others and the ways we are participating in systems of oppression (Loomis, 2011; Zetzer, 2018).

The examination of personal points of privilege, oppression, and discrimination relates to the larger issue of social justice—how we implement personal virtues (e.g., respect, humility, compassion, fairness) and values on a broader scale. Being able to see our privilege—and how we have unknowingly and maybe knowingly contributed to systems of discrimination and oppression—can help us actualize our virtues and values, achieve ethical excellence in our personal and professional lives, and avoid harm to our clients.

We are not suggesting feeling guilty or ashamed of being a White person or having other points of privilege (Spanierman et al., 2009). Rather, we are encouraging you to be aware and to develop understanding about racism and other isms, the cycles of socialization and systems of oppression, and *cultural humility.*

Cultural humility is an attitude and a "way of being" with diverse clients that values the presence and importance of cultural factors (Owen et al., 2011, p. 274) and works toward genuine respect and understanding persons as cultural beings. We might suggest that cultural humility also includes being aware of our privilege and acting to dismantle the systems of oppression in which we have been participating.

Discrimination and Oppression

Discrimination refers to behaviors that usually stem from prejudiced feelings or thoughts and "which denies individuals or groups of people equality of treatment" (Blumenfeld & Raymond, 2000, p. 22). In our opening story, two women of color were both targets of discrimination (not being acknowledged or seen—treated as if they were invisible and denied service) while the White person just behind them was acknowledged and treated respectfully.

The following example is something that happened in Sharon's family some years ago when her children were young and interacted with neighborhood families. The experience addresses another type of privilege and discrimination:

> Bobby (9 years old at the time) said to me (Sharon), "Mom, when we (he and his sister Taya, 8 years old at the time) go over to the neighbor's house to see if Kenny can play, Gene always says, 'Bobby's at the door.' He doesn't say anything about Taya." I asked Bobby why he thought Gene didn't mention Taya when he announced who was at the door. He said he thought it was that Gene didn't like Taya. I responded, "That might be true. It might also be that he doesn't see Taya as 'counting' or deserving notice." The assumption might be that Taya is "invisible" to Gene because of her gender. Whether or not that is Gene's intent, the covert message to Taya may be, "Bobby, you're visible and important to recognize (male privilege) and Taya, you're female; therefore, invisible and don't count."

In all three experiences, the harm was overt and personal. All three individuals were made aware of their "invisibility" by another individual. If we're honest here, there was also some indirect or covert harm that Sharon participated in as she listened to her friend talk about the experience of being invisible at the fast-food restaurant. Sharon initially didn't believe that such a thing could happen—internally discounting her friend's experience of discrimination. Sharon couldn't see her friend's experience of invisibility because of her own unexamined White privilege and resulting participation in systems of oppression. When discrimination takes place on a larger scale, we talk about oppression, which refers to "the systematic, institutionalized mistreatment of one group of people by another" (Lustig & Koester, 1999, p. 159). There is a relationship among discrimination, oppression, and privilege. The equation might look like this: discrimination + privilege (social power) = oppression.

When we become aware of our own points of privilege, we may be able more fully to really hear, empathize with, and respect some of our clients' experiences of discrimination and oppression and thereby acknowledge, rather than discount, their experience (Furman, 2005; Sue et al., 2019; Tuason, 2005).

Journal Entry: *Don't Judge a Book by Its Cover*

Think of a time when you or a person close to you was ignored, devalued, or pre-judged because of age, gender, disability, beliefs (spiritual or political), language or speech, or choice of partner (same gender, skin color difference, another issue of difference). Who was doing the ignoring, devaluing, prejudging? How did it feel? What were the resulting behaviors?

Social Justice

The moral and ethical obligations we have to treat individual people (clients, co-workers, employees, friends, etc.) fairly become more evident with awareness. McIntosh (1990) states it this way: "Describing … privilege makes one newly accountable. As we in women's studies work to reveal male privilege and ask men to give up some of their power, so one who writes about having white privilege must ask, 'Having described it, what will I do to lessen or end it?'" (p. 31).

Recognizing discrimination and our overt or covert participation in oppression because of our points of privilege leads us to considerations of social responsibility and promoting social justice in the profession. Social responsibility has to do with our ethical obligations to help society treat individuals in moral ways—it is a "duty owed to society at large" (Clark, 1993, p. 307) and includes a duty to question and oppose community standards that work against promoting human welfare. Social responsibility means recognizing that societal issues and contexts influence the work in counseling (Sue et al., 2019). With this recognition or understanding, our ethical next step is to social justice counseling/therapy. To provide social justice counseling/therapy might be an opportunity to stretch our core, moral self. There may be clients whose values are very different from ours and our initial thought might be, how can I possibly do good work with someone whose worldview is 180 degrees opposite to mine? Through the lens of social justice, our position is to serve these clients to our best ability (i.e., competence) with respect. We may not agree with them on personal values, needs, and motivations but our position is one of focusing on the client's goals and needs—not what we disagree with from our worldview. Sue et al. (2019) provide us the following definition of social justice counseling/therapy:

> Social justice counseling/therapy is an active philosophy and approach aimed at producing conditions that allow for equal access and opportunity; reducing or eliminating disparities in education, health care, employment, and other areas that lower the quality of life for affected populations; encouraging mental health professionals to consider micro, meso, and macro levels in the assessment, diagnosis, and treatment of clients and client systems. (p. 488)

Hailes et al. (2020) use three domains of justice (interactional, distributive, and procedural) to offer guidelines under each of the domains for us to consider as ways to implement social justice work. The guidelines under interactional justice translate into (a) understanding the relational power dynamics, (b) mitigating those power dynamics, and (c) using approaches that focus on client empowerment and strengths. Power dynamics are inherent in the therapist/client relationship and are complicated by the "intersection of multiple co-occurring identities" that present different amounts of privilege (Hailes et al., p. 3). As psychotherapists we need to be aware of how our identities and interactions within the relationship might reconstruct past experiences of oppression and injustice that our clients from marginalized populations have experienced from others in roles of power and representing institutional power. Among the actions we can take are to (a) elevate collaboration and co-create with clients the goals for therapy, (b) be open to direct communication about perceived assumptions and biases we hold, and (c) draw upon strengths-based approaches which empower clients to "develop their self-advocacy skills, strategies, and resources to be agents of change in their own lives" (p. 4).

Distributive justice focuses on fairness and provision for all, in particular those who have traditionally not received provisions. The specific guidelines include (a) using our energy and resources to serve the main concerns of communities who are marginalized and (b) using our efforts and time to focus on preventive work. Actionable steps could include offering services on a sliding scale, taking on consultant roles in the community for little to no fee, prioritizing preventive or preemptive care to lessen the mental health problems of oppressed groups, and advocacy work to change mental health policies for the better of marginalized populations.

The last domain, procedural justice, includes the last two guidelines: (a) engaging with social systems and (b) raising awareness about system impacts on individual and community wellbeing. The first five guidelines were more on the micro and meso levels; these guidelines tap into the macro level. We can support our clients by getting involved in larger systems that impact them. We might work as allies or advocates in academic settings to provide psychoeducation on matters of oppression and discrimination. We might work with organizations to reform policies within different systems to make them less harmful to marginalized clients.

Understanding our social justice responsibility to our clients and their communities, especially those from marginalized groups, goes beyond the four walls of the therapy room. Sue et al. (2019) suggest we need to expand "the role of the helping professional to include not only counselor/therapist but also advocate, consultant, psychoeducator, change agent, community worker, and so on" (p. 488). Groups of people have been overlooked, devalued, and disrespected because of being different from the "norm" or from the dominant culture (Sue et al., 2019)—including in the world of psychotherapy. As psychotherapists, we are naturally committed to the wellbeing and mental health of our clients. Hopefully, we are also committed to the mental health of the community. We must consider commitment to social justice because the mental health of our clients and community and social justice are inseparably tied together (Hailes et al., 2020).

Journal Entry: *Social Justice and My Core (My Needs, Motivations, and Values)*

The list of social justice counseling roles by Sue and his colleagues may appear daunting to some and exciting to others. You may ask, "How do I perform several roles—such as therapist and advocate or change agent—with my clients and their world? How do these roles even fit together? How does being an advocate, a change agent, or psychoeducator relate to my needs, motivations, and values for being a psychotherapist?"

Take a moment to look back at the exercises in Chapter 1 where you identified or listed your needs and motivations for becoming a psychotherapist and important values for being a psychotherapist. As you review these lists, which needs, motivations, and values suggest a call to promoting or improving the welfare of humans? Which ones are more exclusively individual in nature? Which ones represent a mixed picture—addressing the call to help your individual clients in addition to the call to social justice? Hailes et al. (2020) provided guidelines and actionable items for implementing social justice counseling, and Sue et al. (2019) identified possible roles in social justice counseling/therapy. How do you see yourself as an advocate? consultant? psycho-educator? change agent? community worker? How might you fulfill some of these roles? Which of those struck a chord with your core? What does that say about what's in your core and the foundation for your professional ethical identity?

Closing Thoughts

In this chapter, we've looked at several parts of your core—your moral self. We know that for some readers, this is an uncomfortable chapter to read. Exploring our points of privilege and thinking about how privilege interacts with discrimination and oppression is uncomfortable but necessary work. Let us emphasize four points about this aspect of our mansion and spiral staircase. First, coming to acknowledge our points of privilege is a process, not an event. We've just encouraged you to take the next steps on this journey, but there are always more. Second, all of us have experienced socialization. Thus, we are not alone in this journey. We might have different points of privilege, experience different types of discrimination and oppression, and be at different levels of awareness along the way, but we can certainly benefit from others who are in the process. Third, as soon as we become more aware of how our privilege plays into systems of oppression, we can begin our efforts to be more socially responsible in our work—through entering other roles (i.e., social justice advocate) outside the four walls of psychotherapy. Finally, perfection is not the goal on this journey—but it is an aspiration that motivates us. We encourage you to be willing to have the difficult dialogues, hear the feedback from others (and yourself) along the way, own what is yours. But don't punish yourself for mistakes and missteps along the way.

Understanding privilege, oppression, and social responsibility, along with your values, virtues, motivations, and needs, gives you a firm foundation on which to build your professional ethical identity. We are ready now to explore the ethical acculturation process and the culture of psychotherapy.

3

The Process of Acculturation
Developing Your Professional Ethical Identity

For most of you, the mansion of psychotherapy, and its environment, is very different from your old neighborhood. In fact, it represents a different culture. In this chapter, we discuss the process of moving into the culture of psychotherapy. How do we do that? Let's start with an activity with several scenes and variations. For this activity, we suggest you read all the parts and then respond to aspects of the scenarios and variations that strike you.

Food for Thought: *On the Street Where You Live*

Scenario 1: Imagine that it is a beautiful day. You've launched your new career as a psychotherapist and your case load is growing. Life is good. As you walk down a street not far from where you live, you spot a small group of people coming toward you. You instantly recognize one of the folks; it is Brandon, one of your best friends. Your hand shoots up for a big wave, you smile and call out a friendly "Hello."

Scenario 2: Beautiful day, you've launched your new career, life is good. As you walk down a street not far from where you live, you spot a small group of people coming toward you. You instantly recognize one of the folks as Charlie. In that same split second, you start to smile and lift your hand to wave "Hello" but stop it midair. You stop because Charlie is a client of yours.

In Scenario 1, what went through your mind as you recognized Brandon? What did you think about before you said hello? Was there even the thought not to wave and say hello? What would it have felt like if you had walked by Brandon without saying anything?

In Scenario 2, what went through your mind as you recognized Charlie? What caused you to stop your wave? What are your choices as the two of you walk toward each other on the street?

Variation to Scenario 1: You and Brandon are walking down the street and somebody gives Brandon a big hello. You ask, "Who was that?" In fact, that person was Brandon's therapist but you don't know that. What might happen?

Variation to Scenario 2: Eliza, an acquaintance of yours and another person in the small group, sees you say hello to Charlie. Later that day at a neighborhood get-together, Eliza comes up to you and says, "Charlie is one of my best friends. I didn't know the two of you know each other. How do *you* know Charlie?" How do you respond?

Scenario 3: It is another beautiful day. Your career as a psychotherapist is going well. Your personal life, however, is a different story. You've recently begun working with a psychotherapist. As you're walking down the street, your therapist appears from around the corner. He gives you a big "Hello!" as he walks by. How do you feel? How do you respond?

Variation 1: As he walks away, you hear his walking companion ask him, "Who was that?" How do you feel? How do you hope he responds to the question?

Variation 2: You are walking with a business associate who asks you, "Who was that?" How do you feel? How do you respond?

We assume that in Scenario 1 you had no problem deciding to say hello to your friend. Caring people do that with friends, acquaintances, and sometimes even strangers. However, as a psychotherapist, depending on your context, you have to think more carefully about even these natural social interactions. Here's why: Clients may feel awkward at being greeted by their therapist, and such a greeting may violate *contact confidentiality* (Ahia & Martin, 1993; see Chapter 6). That is, it may communicate to others the private fact that a person is a client.

When we enter the culture of psychotherapy and depending on our practice context, some of these typical human interactions that express our basic needs, motivations, and values don't work the same as in the everyday social interactions we have with our friends. It can be a strange and uncomfortable experience to see somebody on the street with whom we've worked, *intimately* in a therapeutic way, and not acknowledge their existence, even by a wink. This internal discomfort may cause what we will discuss later as *acculturation stress*.

Here's another variation on this story, told by Sharon:

> *We have a counseling lab at Colorado State University for our master's-level students. Our students are recorded working with volunteer clients, most of whom are college students. A couple years ago I'm supervising a student and she's working with this client and they are doing good work. A couple months later, after the semester is over, I see this former client on campus. Immediately I recognize him, but I didn't stop to*

think how I recognize him. I just know that I recognize him. With my friendly side in full gear I say, "Hi." Not just a nondescript "Hi" like I don't know you, but more like, "Hi! How's it goin'?" Then I remember how I know him and realize that he has no clue as to why I am so friendly! In this case, he could be wondering whether I am just an overly friendly person or just downright strange. He had no way of knowing that I had a professional relationship with him as my student's supervisor!

Let's assume that this former client was with a friend and the friend asked, "Who was that?" In this case the former client could genuinely say, "I don't know. Maybe I look like someone else she knows. I've never seen her before." This would be true; he hadn't seen Sharon before. As a supervisor, Sharon had seen a lot of him and knew a lot about his life—from watching the recorded counseling sessions. On the other hand, if Sharon had been this person's therapist and given him that big hello, it could have caused him unnecessary discomfort and embarrassment. He would have three options of how to respond to his friend: choose to tell a lie, choose to tell the truth, or choose to ignore his friend's question. None of these options may feel real good.

One of the costs of being a psychotherapist is having to be more conscious of social interactions. It might mean pausing, even if just for a second, and asking, "How do I know this person?" It might mean being a bit more reserved out in public because we don't know who we might happen to see. We have to take extra steps in situations where other professionals can interact without a second thought. We need to adapt our pre-existing moral sense to the expectations of our new profession. We are not saying that we give up our moral core—those central values that define our morality. Rather, we are saying that we need to pay greater attention to the ethics of our chosen profession, including what that means for our particular practice context.

Of course, many of these types of decisions get easier as we go along. But let's look at another and possibly more conflicted example.

Journal Entry: *Friends and/or Colleagues*

You and your friend both get a job in which you are counseling high school students in an after-school program. The program has a strict policy against drinking or drug use among both students and staff members, and your friend—who is now also your colleague—is showing up for work high.

- How do you feel about your friend's decision to violate the school's policy?
- Do you think you need to report your friend?
  - If yes, why?
  - If no, why not?
- What if you knew that your friend was definitely harming students by coming to work in this condition?

- Would your answer be different from before?
    - If yes, why?
    - If no, why not?
- What values drive your decisions?
- How do you feel about your decisions?
- What if you knew it was mandatory to report this type of behavior by a fellow colleague, would that change your answer?
- If you decided you needed to report your friend, how did you imagine yourself actually taking the necessary steps to action?

Variation: What if the colleague wasn't your friend, just a colleague?

- How do you feel about your colleague's decision?
- Do you decide to report your colleague for violating agency policy?
    - If yes, why?
    - If not, why not?
- What if you knew this person was definitely harming students by coming to work in this condition?
- What values drive your decisions?
- How do you feel about your decisions?
- If you decided you needed to report your colleague, how did you imagine yourself actually taking the necessary steps to action?

There are research data to suggest that both graduate students and practicing psychologists would not behave ethically even when they know they should (Bernard & Jara, 1986; Bernard et al., 1987). It appears as though personal values such as friendship and loyalty get in the way of our professional obligations (Betan & Stanton, 1999), perhaps by making us less objective in our judgments or by weakening our moral courage to uphold our professional responsibility. Whether or not you chose to report your friend's behavior, you might be feeling conflicted, guilty, and/or disloyal. Once again, we need to adapt our pre-existing moral sense to the expectations of our new profession. Let's look more deeply into this process, which we call *ethical acculturation*. Thinking of our professional journey as an acculturation process is like understanding the unique structural qualities of our mansion and the layout of the neighborhood.

The Process of Ethical Acculturation

John Berry and his colleagues (Berry, 1980, 2003; Berry & Kim, 1988; Berry & Sam, 1997) have written extensively about psychological acculturation, the process that immigrants, refugees, sojourners, and others go through when they adapt to a new culture. In this sense, acculturation is defined as "a set of internal psychological out-comes including a clear sense of personal and cultural identity, good mental health, and the achievement of personal satisfaction in the new cultural context" (Berry & Sam, 1997, p. 299). Handelsman et al. (2005) adapted Berry's definition to the notion of ethical acculturation by substituting the word "ethical" for the word "cultural" in this definition.

As we have seen, when we acculturate to the psychotherapy profession we cannot express some of our virtues (e.g., compassion) in the same ways as before. Also, we may have to develop new virtues; for example, virtues surrounding informed consent may include upfront honesty, courage, humility, and what we might call therapeutic informativeness. As Grater (1985) suggested, "To a significant extent the trainee learns to replace social patterns of interacting with therapeutic responses" (p. 606). But the process of acculturation is more compli-cated than merely replacing one set of values, behaviors, or virtues with another. Our pre-existing moral core is not replaced in a wholesale fashion; rather, the best outcome is when what is in our core is refined, adapted, and integrated with the culture of psychotherapy.

Two Dimensions of Acculturation

Berry and Sam (1997) discussed two major dimensions of acculturation: (a) main-tenance and (b) contact and participation. *Maintenance* refers to how much of their culture of origin—the traditions, values, behaviors, language—people bring with them to their new culture. Applied to ethical acculturation, *maintenance* refers to how much of our personal moral sense we bring with us, as it were, to the new culture. As Berry and Sam (1997) state, the task of maintenance is addressed by the person exploring the following question: "Is it considered to be of value to main-tain cultural [ethical, moral] identity and characteristics?" (p. 296). As you review your needs, motivations, values, and virtues—and their expressions—you will notice that some of them you cannot live without, some you can implement in dif-ferent ways, and some (like saying "hello" to everybody you know) might need to be discarded.

Contact and participation, the second dimension, refers to how much we identify with and adopt the traditions, values, behaviors, and language of our new culture. As you deepen your study of psychotherapy, you will discover more and more aspects of the culture that are different from your expectations and, to some extent, different from how you have engaged in relationships before. In the next activity, we give you an opportunity to explore some initial impressions and experiences of entering the psychotherapy culture.

Journal Entry: *Surprise, Surprise*

We've adapted the following questions from Handelsman et al. (2005, p. 62): In studying about your discipline, what is the most counterintuitive, shocking, or surprising professional activity, issue, or value that you have learned about so far? What didn't you expect about being or becoming a psychotherapist? What feelings have you experienced, positively and negatively, about the culture of psychotherapy? You can answer these with general comments, or by telling stories about those times when you felt either that you had signed up for something you didn't bargain for, you felt like you made a mistake, or you simply felt like a stranger in a strange place.

For a few of your observations, you might want to reflect on these questions, which focus on the variables of maintenance as well as contact and participation: What might these surprising elements tell you about the values, traditions, and behaviors involved in psychotherapy? In what ways might these elements be inconsistent with, or discrepant from, your own values and traditions?

Your reflections in this journal entry constitute your knowledge, thus far, of the ethical culture of psychotherapy. Later in this book, we explore the major ethical elements of this culture, such as boundaries, confidentiality, and informed consent.

Four Strategies of Acculturation

If we think of the two dimensions—(a) maintenance and (b) contact and participation—as variables along which one can be relatively high or low, we see the possibility of four alternatives for acculturation choices. We can be high on both maintenance and contact, low on both dimensions, or high on one and low on the other (see Figure 3.1). "*Attitudes* towards these four alternatives, and actual *behaviors* exhibiting them, together constitute an individual's acculturation *strategy*" (Berry & Sam, 1997, p. 297, emphases in original). Let's take a look at each of the four types of strategies applied to ethical acculturation.

Integration

When we desire to hold onto our core and engage with the professional culture, and our behaviors reflect both our moral core and the ethical values of psychotherapy, we are choosing the strategy of integration. Integration can occur in different ways,

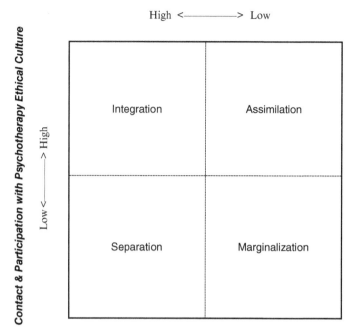

Figure 3.1 Strategies of Ethical Acculturation. (Adapted from Handelsman et al., 2005)

including: (a) upholding a personal value that overlaps with a professional value; (b) modifying the expression of a personal value; (c) creating and internalizing a new value; and/or (d) reorganizing or reprioritizing our values. The following paragraphs illustrate each of these options.

Sometimes an integration strategy involves a relatively simple overlapping of our moral core with the values of the professional culture. For example, we may hold this value: "When people we care about are in distress, we give them our undivided attention." This value works for our close friends, professional colleagues, and psychotherapy clients.

However, because psychotherapy is a unique kind of relationship, a simple overlap of values and their expression is less frequent than we might think. Integration more often means that we need to modify the expression of existing values. In addition, we make some of these modifications based on context and cultural considerations. For example, when we see a client walking down the street toward us we need to consider the best ways to demonstrate respect. Sometimes that respect might look like a slight acknowledgement and nothing more. In other contexts, it might mean that we acknowledge them and even stop to talk just briefly while still maintaining the confidentiality of the relationship. We have thus upheld the personal value of respect and the professional value of confidentiality (among others).

Another example of modifying the expression of values concerns privacy, which we discuss in detail in Chapter 6. With our friends, we respect their privacy by not talking about them to strangers, but it may be perfectly acceptable to talk about our friends to our spouses, partners, or closest friends. However, when the personal value of privacy is integrated with the professional value of confidentiality, we refrain from talking about our clients to *anybody*, even our partners, closest friends, and relatives.

A third example of modifying our expression of values might be how and if and when we give advice. Giving advice to friends might be an expression of our concern and compassion. In psychotherapy, however, depending on the context and the client's cultural background, we are working to encourage the client to gather good information, deliberate, and then make decisions. In the psychotherapy relationship, demonstrating concern and compassion might mean giving less advice, or different kinds of advice. (We will revisit issues around giving advice in Chapter 5.)

As we can see, sometimes integration means adapting our behavior to express pre-existing values in a new context. However, at other times we need to create and internalize entirely new values. For some of us, privacy is not really an issue among friends. We might have a circle of friends and it is perfectly acceptable to talk within that circle about any of the conversations we have with any of our friends. In the psychotherapy culture, we need an entirely new concept of privacy and confidentiality: In the psychotherapy relationship, the information clients share with you is *not* yours to disclose outside of the relationship. The ownership of clients' information remains with clients, who must give permission, barring any exceptions to confidentiality addressed in Chapter 6, for you to share it with anybody else.

Another new concept in the psychotherapy profession to which we need to adapt concerns being honest or sharing information about what we do and who we are. In psychotherapy, this is called *informed consent* (see Chapter 7). In friendship, we typically do not ask explicit permission of people to become their friend but discover how important it is to be honest and oneself as the relationship grows. However, in psychotherapy the process is different. There is a kind of laying all the cards out on the table—via the informed consent process—where we share information about ourselves as a professional and ask clients explicitly if they wish to become our clients.

Another variation of the integration strategy is to reorganize our values—we elevate the relative importance of some of our values or create a higher value that helps us adapt to our psychotherapeutic roles. Take a moment and go back to take a look at your values lists from Chapter 1. You might have identified loyalty and compassion to be among your highest values—after all, they are key elements of a good friendship. Loyalty and compassion in friendship involve such behaviors as self-disclosure, saying hello when you meet your friend on the street, lending or receiving money when either of you are in need, or being your friend's first insurance client.

As a professional psychotherapist however, your implementation of values such as loyalty and compassion will revolve around confidentiality, consent, and maintaining boundaries that benefit our clients. Your implementation will depend upon your practice context and your clientele. However, it's a pretty safe bet that demonstrating these values will involve less self-disclosing to clients, *not* entering into business arrangements with clients, and *not* doing therapy with those with whom you have another relationship. With all these constraints, we might conclude that to be a therapist means not showing or experiencing compassion. If this thought has crossed your mind, you might be thinking, "What am I doing in this profession? I am all about people and being compassionate."

The solution to this dilemma—or acculturation crisis (Berry & Kim, 1988)—is realizing that the integration strategy doesn't negate the value of compassion; rather, it encourages us to put the value of *respect* at the top of our values hierarchy in our professional life. Knowing we are upholding the value of respect allows us to retain a sense of consistency across situations—although showing respect may need to look somewhat different depending on the practice context and the people with whom we work. Integration strategies help us recognize and reduce the tension between our personal and professional roles and identities. Integration means that we can read the ethical standards of our profession and think, "I understand the values behind the rules and I can heartily endorse those values. I'll find ethical ways to deal with the inevitable tension between any of my personal values and those of my new profession."

In terms of psychological acculturation, Berry and his colleagues conclude, "Evidence strongly supports a positive correlation between the use of this strategy and good psychological adaptation during acculturation" (Berry & Sam, 1997, p. 298). We believe that making the effort to integrate our personal and professional ethics will lead to good *ethical* adaptation, which gives us the best chance of becoming and staying ethically excellent psychotherapists.

Before we leave this section on integration, we need to make two points very clear. First, integration does not mean bending the rules to fit our personal needs, motivations, or values. It also doesn't involve simply splitting the difference between your core and the professional identity you are nurturing. Rather, integration has more to do with how we approach professional rules. Now that you have explored what is in your core, you are able to explore how you fit with the profession, what it means to be you in the profession, and how best to serve clients, students, consultees, and the broader society.

Second, even when we use integration strategies and we behave in ethically excellent ways, it might not always feel good—it might actually feel uncomfortable! The joy and fulfillment of behaving ethically is sometimes overshadowed by unpleasantness engendered by what philosophers call the wrong-making features (Ross, 1930/1998) of many actions—those aspects that are not ethically perfect because of values conflicts or other considerations. For example, when we report colleagues for unprofessional behavior we feel angry at the position they put us in and sad that their careers and relationships may suffer. We may also feel conflicted when we've behaved consistently with our profession even as we are aware of our limitations: not being able to help as much as we'd like, not being able to fully pursue our interests, and so forth. For example, we might be convinced that entering into a business partnership with a client would be beneficial to everyone involved, but we know that this would be an unethical multiple relationship (see Chapter 5).

Assimilation

We might believe that being a psychotherapist is *so* different from any other role we play that we might as well build our professional self from scratch. Thus, we might actively jettison, or simply lose track of, our own moral sense and we totally adopt the ethical values and traditions of psychotherapy as our sole source of professional guidance. This is an extreme of the strategy of *assimilation*.

You might be thinking, "What's wrong with assimilation? Aren't I supposed to follow the rules of the profession?" To those of you thinking this, we applaud your motivation and your dedication to the profession. Indeed, to the observer, many assimilation behaviors would look identical to integration behaviors. However, just following the rules to the letter is not enough to be an ethical professional. Advanced degrees, professional licenses, nicely furnished offices, and business attire do not make a professional ethical. "These outward signs are meaningless and potentially harmful without a firm personal grounding in and appreciation for the ethics and value traditions of the professional culture" (Handelsman et al., 2005, p. 61). As Blasi stated, our ethical ideals are "powerless if they are not rooted in a moral self" (1984, p. 130).

In the short term, assimilation strategies might be appropriate until we gain more knowledge about ourselves in the profession and can move toward integration. For example, it is a good idea, as a new psychotherapist, to maintain client confidentiality even if you don't yet really grasp the connection between that behavior and your own moral sense. However, if you maintain this strategy over time you might become alienated from the profession, like you are just going through the motions, because you are following rules without engaging your core. The rules become hollow because you feel little or no personal investment in either the rules or their underlying values. As ethical decisions become more difficult (remember the journal entry with your hypothetical friend/colleague using drugs), you may find it harder to make the subtle judgments or implement the uncomfortable choices that are required. Another risk is that your new professional sensibilities will spill over into your non-therapy relationships. You may find, for example, that you feel the need to recommend or provide professional help to every person in your social circles, especially your family members and close friends. This is an indication that you have lost yourself in the acculturation process.

Consider this scenario: You come home from a day of therapy and your spouse or partner asks, "How'd it go today?" You know that you are supposed to keep client information confidential and you are determined to obey that rule so you reply,

"I'm sorry, I'm not allowed to say." Your partner responds, "But I'm your partner; we share our lives with each other! Don't you want to remain close?" And they have a point! If you choose an extreme assimilation strategy, you might hold your ground and refuse to discuss your work at all. But this response is based on a skewed, half-informed understanding of the rules and their applications.

In contrast, an integration strategy might lead you to keep in mind the rules about confidentiality but also appreciate your values about close human relationships. Thus, you might choose to share some of your feelings without violating client confidentiality: "Well, the day started well; my first couple of sessions felt really good and this was rewarding—like I really got a chance to do what I was trained to do. But in the afternoon I struggled more in my sessions. I was pretty frustrated by the end of the day." Notice that your partner will not know who your clients are or about the clients' part of the therapy, but can stay in touch with who *you* are and how the day was.

We hope this scenario illustrates our point that integration does not mean bending the rules; rather, true integration into the professional culture has to do with how we draw upon our core to handle the rules. Observers may not be able to tell if we're using assimilation or integration strategies, because from the outside they might look like identical adherence to the rules. The differences will be internal; therapists choosing integration strategies have found areas of overlap between what they value, who they are personally, and what they must do professionally. They feel more comfortable with the tensions that may exist between these two spheres, and may be more able to choose and implement ethical excellence.

Separation

If we choose to look for ethical guidance only in our moral core, and do not identify with the culture of psychotherapy, we are choosing the strategy of separation. Many beginning students of psychotherapy choose separation strategies in their ethical deliberations because they do not yet know about the culture of therapy (see Chapter 4). They are relying on their personal frameworks for how relationships work and/or see the rules as limiting or confining. They have not yet begun to see the ethical rules as grounded in ethical principles that provide a firm foundation for ethical choices.

Again, imagine being at the dinner table with your partner, who asks you how it went today. You feel that unburdening yourself after a difficult day would be a mentally healthy thing to do. It would make you feel better. It would even help you get back into the office tomorrow and have a better day. Indeed, you'd be a better therapist! So you start,

> David and Eleanor's sessions went quite well. You remember Eleanor—she's the accountant who was getting anxious about her upcoming exams? Thank goodness, she's doing much better. But in the afternoon, Alan's session was

tough. He works downtown, you know, where our insurance woman's office is—the next office. Anyway, his daughter Sarah isn't doing well at school. Sarah just started Rutland Elementary School, where our Jason's going to go next year …

You feel so much better after sharing about your whole day. In addition, you are sure your clients wouldn't mind you talking about them to your partner because, after all, it's really for their own benefit.

In this situation, you are using a separation strategy. You are acting only from your pre-existing moral sense (Kitchener & Anderson, 2011), including doing good for clients based only on your own moral guides and conception of relationships. You feel like you are handling your partnership well because you value sharing in the relationship, you see your conversation as a way of taking care of yourself, and your intention may be to help your clients by debriefing the day in a caring relationship. However, in making these decisions, you are not valuing the demands of the professional principle of confidentiality and the client's right to privacy. Despite your good intentions, you may actually be doing harm. Your behaviors violate the privacy of your client and are unethical.

Separation may also show itself when the personal values of clients conflict with your own values and needs. For example, family members, friends, financial planners, religious advisors, and others may not have any prohibitions against condemning their friends' or clients' plans to get a divorce, have an affair, marry a person with another skin color, vote Libertarian, marry their childhood sweetheart, not have children, buy an extended warranty on their car, or listen to jazz. However, the profession expects therapists not to impose personal values and needs on their clients. Put in simple terms: Your task as a therapist is to encourage clients to live the life they want and need to live themselves, not the life you want for them.

Bucher and Stelling (1977) conducted a longitudinal study of professional training programs in internal medicine, psychiatry, and biochemistry. They discussed what they called *socialization failures*—students who did not fit the mold of the training program. Among the characteristics of these socialization failures was a rigid commitment to a pre-existing value orientation. We might guess that these students adopted separation strategies, and although they have had good intentions for their future profession, they never identified with their new professional cultures. It is important to realize that good intentions are not enough to assure good professional practice. As Handelsman et al. (2005) said:

> Although they may have a very strong personal code of ethics and be very well intentioned, these students may also be unaware of the potential harm that may come from acting on a set of principles or virtues that are inconsistent with the professional context. (p. 61)

In light of this discussion, it might appear that ethical rules may take away some of the choices we thought we had. When you run across ethical standards that don't strike you as right or beneficial to the client, you may think of them as stupid little rules or barriers to effective work and therefore not necessary to follow. Edging toward integration, however, means that we appreciate that the consistency that ethical rules and guidelines provide helps us treat clients ethically. This consistency actually provides the necessary conditions under which we can learn about and empathize with the uniqueness of our clients. If your first reaction is to minimize the importance of the ethical guidelines, we would encourage you to think of professional rules in these ways:

- Perhaps they are professional implementations of higher values that you actually have in common with the culture of psychotherapy.
- They are an opportunity for you to see if you can articulate your own values, virtues, motivations, and needs along with the values, traditions, and principles that underlie the standard. Then, you are on your way to integrating who you are at your core with the culture of psychotherapy.
- They are, ironically perhaps, the key to your future fulfillment as an ethically excellent psychotherapist! If followed from true understanding and appreciation they will produce ethical excellence. They are an opportunity to explore a positive ethical approach: You can take the opportunity to see how you can achieve higher purposes by going beyond what the rule says as the minimum. Here's an example: Some states require informing clients that sex between clients and therapists is a crime. At the very least, you could reproduce the statute in your informed consent statement (see Chapter 7) and ask the client to read it and sign a document that they have read the relevant statute. Or you could use this "disclosure rule" as a stimulus to talk with clients about a range of topics, including a variety of the boundaries of the therapy relationship (see Chapter 5).

Marginalization

Marginalization is the worst of both worlds. "Those exhibiting marginalization will obey ethical standards out of personal convenience rather than a sense of moral commitment" (Handelsman et al., 2005, p. 61). We neither identify with our new culture nor are we solidly grounded in our own moral core. Marginalization is similar to a rudderless ship on the sea—drifting along with no mechanism to guide its course (Gilley et al., 2008).

Marginalization can be a temporary strategy. We may begin our training thinking that we can simply adopt a professional persona, but we are still unaware of what the new culture entails. As a result, we make mistakes, like suggesting specific courses of action for our clients simply because they're expedient or would somehow benefit us, or being so stiff and serious with a client that we don't make a connection.

Sometimes we may get dislodged from our moral compasses when we are impaired in some way. Going through a divorce or other relationship crisis, losing support groups when we move, or abusing drugs or alcohol are all examples of times when we might choose marginalization. We might falsify work records to secure more money, or we might "judge" that it's best for a couple we are seeing to split up, secretly hoping that this could lead to a social or romantic relationship with one member of the couple. These are behaviors that are clearly wrong professionally, and we hope you would judge them as wrong according to your own moral core and your growing professional ethical identity.

Journal Entry: *Acculturation Strategies*

As you were reading about the acculturation strategies, you might have thought, "Wow, I remember when I …" or "You know, now I understand why …" In this entry, write down some of those thoughts. Try to think of times when your behavior or attitude (or the behavior or attitude of someone you observed) demonstrates each one of the four strategies.

We imagine that you will be (or have been) a psychotherapist who strives to choose integration strategies and succeeds most of the time. However, there will be times when you will not choose integration. When that's the case, which strategy are you most likely to choose? Are you most likely to slip into assimilation strategies (e.g., "Let me just follow the rules to protect myself even though I really don't see the value"); separation strategies (e.g., "I'm a nice person, so what I do will naturally be therapeutic"); or marginalization strategies (e.g., "What's the use of even trying to do the right thing?")?

Acculturation Stress

Acculturation stress refers to the difficulties we may face as we adapt to being a psychotherapist. As we've touched on earlier, acculturation stress can arise when our response as a professional needs to be different than that as a friend.

Acculturation stress can start early in our careers. For example, one source of stress is that the culture of psychotherapy and your training are imperfect. You may find, for example, that your professors, supervisors, and others you thought would be perfect role models may not be so perfect (Branstetter & Handelsman, 2000; Glaser & Thorpe, 1986; Hammel et al., 1996).

Another example of acculturation stress: Not every professional you meet will be comfortable talking about ethical issues. Here are just two cases. Some psychotherapists find it difficult to admit to others that they have had sexual feelings for clients (see Pope et al., 2006). Other psychotherapists may be quick to interpret a question about their ethics as an accusation of misbehavior and they may experience your inquiry about the ethical rationale for their behavior as an ethical insult (Veatch & Sollitto, 1976).

In addition, you may also find that psychotherapy does not help all who seek services, or not to the extent you would like. It may be a new realization for you that problems for which people seek psychotherapy are not easily solved! Some clients, for example, will have thought of virtually all of the solutions that occur to you and already have many reasons why such solutions won't work.

Food for Thought: *Acculturation Stress*

Imagine the following scenario: The clinical director of the mental health center calls and offers you a job. She mentions that the clincher for her in you getting the job was your comment about wanting to help people since you were very young. You are confident that you will do well, but even so you are a little nervous. The night before your first day on the job you dream about the most unpleasant type of person you've ever known or heard about. This person triggers feelings of anger and disgust any time you think about them. The next day, your very first client is a person who in some important ways reminds you of the person in your dream. They look like the person, they're a member of the same group as the person, and they have the same attitudes. What do you think? How do you feel? What are your options? What would you do if you had no constraints? What do you do?

Now put yourself in the role of the client, and the therapist has these feelings toward you. What are you expecting from this therapist? How would you react if they did what you were considering as the therapist?

Acculturation stress can also involve a mismatch between your strengths and the skills required of a psychotherapist. These are inevitable because no one person can ever master all the skills involved in all types of psychotherapy with all types of clients. For example, you may be a problem-solver by nature and feel impatient with friends and colleagues who like to mull over options, reflect, and deliberate before taking action. Your problem-solving approach may work very well in your social relationships, in your other jobs (as a stockbroker, ski instructor, software developer), and with your recreational activities. In psychotherapy, quick problem-solving is the exception rather than the rule; you may find yourself challenged to expand your repertoire of helping behaviors and attitudes.

The gulf between the skills, virtues, values, and motivations you bring and those required of psychotherapists is similar to what Berry and Sam (1997) called *cultural distance* (p. 307). If the distance between the two cultures, in this case your ethical traditions and those of psychotherapy, is very great, you may need to engage in some *cultural shedding*, which Berry and Sam defined as "the *un*learning of aspects of one's previous repertoire that are no longer appropriate" (p. 298).

If you are coming into the psychotherapy profession after having been in another profession, such as law, medicine, or even other mental health activities, your cultural shedding may be especially stressful. You may find that skills you thought would be helpful are not. Handelsman et al. (2005) present the following example:

> One trainee had previously worked as a counselor in a domestic abuse shelter, where it was common for counselors to engage in substantial self-disclosure, especially about their own abuse backgrounds. She initially resented the admonition that her self-disclosures as a psychologist had to be more selective and carefully timed. (p. 63)

Coming from other professions may also be stressful because of the loss of status, power, or prestige. As Berry and Kim (1988) state: "One's 'entry status' into the larger society [psychotherapy] is often lower than one's 'departure status' from the home society" (p. 216).

Trying to understand ethical standards which often appear (or are) vague and contradictory can prompt acculturation stress. When our students have asked for an answer to an ethical issue, on more than one occasion we've responded with, "It depends." This ambiguity or seeming contradictions are one of the most frustrating features of the profession for many of our students. For example, psychotherapists are required to maintain confidentiality but also to report child abuse. In addition, psychotherapists are required to report their clients' threats of physical harm against others, but not report the fact that a client has committed a crime in the past (see Chapter 6). At these times, the stress we face may feel really awful. "If conflict and tension do appear, a highly stressful *crisis* phase may then occur, in which the conflict comes to a head, and a resolution is required" (Berry & Kim, 1988, p. 210).

Acculturation Stress in Professional and Personal Relationships

Acculturation is an all-encompassing phenomenon, not just a professional one. To begin this discussion, let's do some reflecting.

Food for Thought: *More Acculturation Stress*

Think about some of the circumstances in your life that have changed along with entering a psychotherapy training program. These circumstances can be economic changes; less family and other support; attitude changes toward you among your friends and relations; or adjustments you've had to make to a new set of friends, professors, colleagues, and so forth. What would make some of these stresses easier? What types of circumstances would be too stressful for you?

The acculturation process changes both our professional relationships and our personal ones. By adopting new values and reorienting the ones we have, we inevitably make and experience shifts in our personal relationships. These shifts also occur because people treat us differently. The uncomfortable news is that people close to us may struggle with the change. On the other hand, changes in both types of relationships can be quite positive. With the broader perspective that comes from integration, we may find that we can develop a range of skills that are helpful in all our relationships.

Food for Thought: *Acculturating to Using Social Media as a Professional*

Imagine this scenario: You make a new friend, and one afternoon you have finished work a little early. You have Google open already, and just before you close it you enter your new friend's name—perhaps just to see if they're on Facebook or LinkedIn. Or to see if what they said about their employment, or the part of town they live in, was true. Or because you think this is a relationship that might go somewhere. You google them, find out that there's nothing much beyond what they told you, and you close up your laptop for the night (or the next 15 minutes). Nobody, neither your new friend nor your old friends, knows.

What would have happened if you DID find something *interesting* about your new friend? How comfortable would you feel, the next time you met them, to say, "You know, I googled you, and what you said the last time we met wasn't quite true, was it?" Would you want to tell your other friends about what you found?

Let's dig a little deeper, change up the scenario a couple more times, and see if these change anything:

You are a therapist, and your new "friend" is not a friend but a new client. How might that change the scenarios?

Now, imagine the story is about your therapist, and *you* are the new client. Would that change what you'd like the therapist in the scenarios to do?

Authors are using the term *patient-targeted googling* (PTG; Reinert & Kowacs, 2019) to describe the practice of getting information about patients from social media. We explore confidentiality and other ethical principles relevant to PTG later. For now, we want to illustrate the point that the deliberations you undertake and the choices you make in personal versus professional situations are different, and may lead to acculturation stress.

One source of stress in this situation is that the profession is still deciding how it feels about PTG (Asay & Lal, 2014). Attitudes toward PTG are all over the place, with studies showing both approval (Eichenberg & Herzber, 2016) and disapproval (DiLillo & Gale, 2011). PTG may be more appropriate in some situations than in others (Ashby et al., 2015), and the ethical issues are varied and complex (Reinert & Kowacs, 2019).

What are your personal values and practices about "friend-targeted googling"? How might those pre-existing values about social media influence your reactions to arguments for and against PTG?

How to Deal with Acculturation Stress

Keep Learning

Remember that learning to become ethically excellent is not an event that happens in 10 or 16 weeks; rather, it is a life-long process (Handelsman, 2001b). Ethical acculturation never stops! Over the course of your professional life, you will change and the professional culture will change. For example, it wasn't that long ago when managed care didn't exist, teletherapy didn't exist, Prozac didn't exist, and even family therapy didn't exist. We encourage you to be open to exploration of yourself and the profession.

Keep Your Eyes Open

You may start with simple notions, but don't stop there. For example, "Put your clients' needs above your own" is a nice platitude to keep in mind, but reality happens. Something's gotta give when your client calls in crisis and needs to see you and at the same time you are sitting in the emergency room receiving area with your sick child. Remember that psychotherapy, ethics, clients and their problems, and you and your life are more complex than it might first appear.

Keep Your Mind Open

If you are not "getting it" when your professors, supervisors, or colleagues talk with you about ethical requirements, do not immediately assume that you are an unethical person or cannot become an ethical therapist. At the same time, don't assume that your professors and supervisors are totally off the wall. We encourage you to take some time to think through the acculturation stress you are facing and explore a variety of avenues that will help you choose integration strategies. Find some very good ethical role models and see what they have to offer. Be especially cognizant of their advice when you feel most stressed. But keep your eyes open and remember that nobody's perfect.

Keep Your Mouth Open!

You should develop an ethical support network of professors, colleagues, fellow students, and even folks in other professions. The more you can get into the habit of seeing the professional world in terms of ethics, the smoother your acculturation will be.

Keep Your Heart Open

Give yourself some time to develop a full range of ethical reasoning and reflecting skills. Strive for perfection, but don't be too hard on yourself when it doesn't quite happen. Keep a sense of perspective and strive to become more fully human as you become more fully professional.

Mismatch with the Profession?

As we were writing this first part of the book, we talked a lot about having a section that raises the possibility that psychotherapy may not be the profession for you. We questioned ourselves about where and how to address the issue. We decided to be honest and not pull any punches. After all, taking a positive approach doesn't mean that everything will be wonderful. Thus, as we end this chapter we plant a seed: Being honest about yourself means that you need to consider the possibility that the outcome of your journey will be a decision that you will *not* become a psychotherapist.

What Sharon says to her graduate classes is this: "Not everybody who applies to be in a counseling program should be in a counseling program. It just isn't the right niche for them." So, we'd like to give you a place to back out gracefully. There might be professions that better match with your ethical core. You may find that there aren't enough professional or personal motivations that can satisfy you as a therapist. The overlap between your personal motivations and values on the one hand and the values and motives expected of a therapist on the other may be small. You may find that there are other professions, or other professional activities, that will suit you better. It's OK to do so. It's OK to recognize that "this is not the profession for me." That's a good decision, an ethical decision.

By the way, this realization can also happen for people who have been working happily and effectively as psychotherapists for years. Life changes, people change, the profession changes. The journey is ongoing. Different priorities come up. Some therapists find a time in their careers when they say, "I need a change. This is not working for me anymore."

If you decide that being a psychotherapist is not right for you, it doesn't necessarily mean that you become a salesperson, talk show host, or professional wrestler. You may still become a counselor, social worker, or psychologist who does different activities, like assessment, consultation, or research.

Here's a related example from Sharon:

> My financial planner's associate has his doctorate in psychology. I found this information very interesting so I asked about the switch. He said that soon after his internship he decided that psychology was not what he wanted to do. He really likes working with people and he likes research and assessment, but he wanted a different context for these personal values and motivations. So when we're talking about my financial strategies, he goes back to the psychology literature to back up his points. What's intriguing to me is that he went through an entire doctoral program, he had the presence of mind and judgment to know it wasn't going to work for him, and he had the courage to make the switch.

We also decided to tell you that the two of us spend almost no time doing psychotherapy at this point in our careers. We write, consult, teach, administer, and train. We've both been psychotherapists at times in our lives and there may be times in the future when we do therapy again. At this point, helping you become an ethical therapist fulfills our values and motivations of helping students become ethically excellent therapists.

4

Navigating the Ethical Culture of Psychotherapy

Mitch remembers a student in his ethics course who became discouraged with all the bad stuff that the class was discussing: therapists having sex with clients, defrauding insurance companies, violating confidentiality, and doing all kinds of other unethical things. She also started to think that she might not have the natural ability to become a good, ethical therapist. As Mitch and the student discussed her feelings, it became clearer that she was having an acculturation crisis. The field of psychotherapy, she was learning, was much more than having clients come in with problems and therapists providing solutions. The skills involved in being a psychotherapist include, but are much more than, naturally occurring abilities and tendencies. In addition, the ethical dimensions of the profession and the skills necessary to appreciate those ethical dimensions are not usually intuitive.

Mitch's student was standing at the entrance to the mansion. She might have felt uncomfortable with her motivations, her moral core, or her level of self-care, all of which we've explored with you so far. She might (also) have felt intimidated about the adventures before her: the nature of the mansion and its neighborhood, the steepness or complexity of the spiral staircases, or the darkness in some parts of the building. Our purpose in this chapter is to make the process of entering and navigating your new professional edifice more manageable. We will provide some ethical foundations, some guides, and some specifics about tripping points and how to recognize them.

So far, we've encouraged you to take stock of your "culture of origin" using an ethical lens. Now it is time to focus on the culture of psychotherapy to which you have been adapting. If you are a seasoned therapist, you will have much to reflect upon, including the changes you have seen in the professional culture over time. If you are a newcomer, however, you may be more able to identify the specific aspects of this new culture that are unexpected or that take some time to acclimate to.

Regardless of where you are—on your way to the mansion, moving in, or helping to renovate—you most likely have been or will be frustrated at times. We routinely encounter frustration and sometimes anger in our students, trainees, and workshop participants, who want us to just tell them "the answer" to an ethical dilemma. This is a very common part of ethical acculturation. The good news about this situation is that the frustration is a natural byproduct of learning such lessons as (a) not all ethical situations have clear answers, (b) it takes concentrated effort to resolve ethical dilemmas, (c) the profession they are entering is a complex one, and (d) making and doing the ethical choice doesn't always *feel* good.

Guides to Acting Ethically

Wouldn't it be nice if therapists could or should simply be really nice people who have some good motivations and virtues? However, because of the complexity of psychotherapy and because of the high stakes and risk of harm, even the most virtuous people need additional ethical guidance when they become professional therapists. This is where professional ethics come in.

Every major mental health organization has a code of professional ethics (e.g., American Association for Marriage and Family Therapy, 2015; American Counseling

Table 4.1 Ethical Foundations for Psychotherapists.

Ethical Foundations

1. **Do good** or seek to benefit clients and prospective clients. The ethical principle of *beneficence*.
2. **Avoid doing harm** or exploiting clients. The ethical principle of *nonmaleficence*.
3. **Respect clients' autonomy**—their freedom of action and freedom of choice. The ethical principle of *respect for autonomy*.
4. **Treat clients fairly**. The ethical principle of *justice*.
5. Embrace our **social responsibility**. The ethical principle of *social justice*, or *general beneficence* (Knapp et al., 2017).
6. Be **trustworthy**, faithful, and loyal to clients by keeping promises. The ethical principle of *fidelity*.
7. **Speak the truth** to clients and potential clients. The ethical principle of *veracity*.
8. These are not principles, but we want to remind you to **cultivate virtues**, including
   - Honesty
   - Humility
   - Diligence
   - Prudence
   - Integrity

Sometimes these foundational principles and virtues can conflict with each other.

There are other guides that are a bit more specific that we can add to this list:

- Become and remain competent.
- Pursue your interests without conflicts, or minimizing the effects of them.
- Respect clients' privacy.
- Continue to develop your cultural competence.
- Inform clients of important information, and get their consent to treatment.
- Maintain your professional boundaries.

Association, 2014; American Psychological Association, 2017; Canadian Psychological Association, 2017; National Association of Social Workers, 2017). The different codes of ethics vary, but they share many elements, including what we call the *Ethical Foundations for Psychotherapists* (see Table 4.1). These statements highlight the ethical values in the culture of psychotherapy and act as basic guides for choosing and evaluating behavior.

As you consider the Ethical Foundations in Table 4.1, notice three things. First, we've worded them all in as positive a way as possible. Second, they are not answers! Rather, they are guides. Many organizations supplement their ethics codes with more specific statements of professional standards. (You can find links to more than 40 statements of ethical standards and practice guidelines at http://kspope.com/ethcodes/index. php.) However, no ethical principle or standard can provide specific answers for all the situations therapists may face. Third, the guides might conflict with each other in practice because of the complexity of the choices therapists need to make.

Journal Entry: *Foundations*

Take a moment and reflect (in writing) on each one of the Ethical Foundations. See if you can recall or speculate about one example of something therapists can do to follow or exemplify each Foundation, and one example of something therapists can do that would violate the Foundation.

Psychotherapy Is a Unique Relationship

We need these guides because the psychotherapy relationship—perhaps more than any other professional relationship—is both very potent and very fragile. By potent we mean that it has the potential to enhance clients' lives and help them grow. By fragile we mean that the relationship is delicate and easily contaminated. Handling this relationship with care—to maximize benefits and minimize harms and risks—is one of our most fundamental responsibilities as therapists.

Psychotherapists come from a multitude of programs. These cover disciplines such as psychology, counseling, social work, family therapy, psychiatry, and several newer fields. No matter the context in which psychotherapy is taught and learned, all therapeutic relationships share some essential features, which we list now and then explore in some detail:

- The psychotherapy relationship includes professional care and concern—and it is not a "friendship."
- The therapy relationship is complex in terms of power.
- The general goal is for clients to be better after having experienced the relationship than before.
- Within the relationship, psychotherapists offer skill and expertise.
- Trust is the foundation upon which the therapeutic relationship rests.
- Therapists have ethical and legal responsibilities to clients.

The Therapeutic Relationship Comprises Professional Care and Concern

We might be helpful to others in many types of relationships, yet the therapy relationship requires a unique kind of care and concern. As such, it is different from friendship, with which most of us have much experience. Psychotherapists, in contrast to friends, provide a different kind of human connection. For example, psychotherapists are there to work hard for and be there for clients—but not the other way around. The therapeutic relationship is asymmetrical; you cannot and should not expect the same kind of care and concern *from* your clients as you provide *to* your clients. (We talk more about this in Chapter 5.)

Therapy Represents a Complex Power Relationship

As psychotherapists, we are experts in human behavior and change, but we are not exclusively responsible for clients making changes or taking on new behaviors. The control over what happens in therapy, and to some extent the growth of clients, we share with clients in our professional role—although in a complicated way. For example: Clients have the power to decide whether to enter therapy, yet both therapists and clients share decision making about the therapeutic goals and some of the general strategies. Therapists decide how to apply therapeutic techniques, yet clients make the decision whether to use or not use what they gain from therapy in their day-to-day lives. Both clients and psychotherapists decide whether therapy is working well enough to continue, yet clients ultimately decide whether they have met their goals and whether to continue with or to end therapy. (See Chapter 9 for a fuller discussion of termination issues.)

The General Goal Is for Clients to Be Better After Experiencing the Relationship

Psychotherapists work to make their relationship with clients functional and healthy, with clarified boundaries and expectations. Through this healthy relationship, clients have the opportunity to see what good communication and respectful boundaries look and feel like. When therapists keep their personal needs out of the relationship and keep clients' needs first, clients will likely leave the relationship in better psychological health.

Within the Relationship, Psychotherapists Offer Skill and Expertise

When clients purchase psychotherapy, they are really purchasing therapists' expertise and its appropriate use. Expertise is a hallmark of a profession (Cruess et al., 2004). Consequently, psychotherapists have certain professional obligations, including knowing about how the therapeutic relationship works, understanding the dynamics of change and growth, knowing how to think about problems and their solutions, and recognizing the limits of their own professional competence.

Trust Is the Foundation upon Which the Therapeutic Relationship Rests

For good work to happen in therapy, clients need to trust their therapist in at least four ways:

1. Clients need to trust that psychotherapists have the requisite knowledge to help them.
2. Clients need to trust that psychotherapists are *using* their skills and knowledge in beneficial ways.
3. Clients need to trust that psychotherapists will be diligent and work hard with them in the therapy process.
4. Clients need to trust that their wellbeing is the utmost priority in the therapy. As we explored in the previous chapter, this does not mean that therapists cannot meet any of their own needs. It does mean, however, that getting these needs met should not come at the expense of clients' wellbeing and goal attainment.

Therapists Have Ethical and Legal Responsibilities

Ethical principles and values underlie every aspect of psychotherapy. For example, the principle of beneficence—our Foundation #1 about doing good—justifies the existence of the entire psychotherapy profession. It also means doing an excellent job by keeping in mind why the relationship is there in the first place. Ethics provides a positive base for our work that can help us work toward ethical excellence and avoid problems and complaints.

In addition to ethical responsibilities, therapists have legal responsibilities to clients. Because the therapeutic relationship is fragile and therapists can exploit and harm clients, states and provinces regulate many of the professions that practice psychotherapy. Regulations identify therapists' obligations and clarify legal protections for clients. For example, many state and provincial laws recognize the psychotherapy relationship as a privileged relationship (see Chapter 6), similar to the doctor–patient relationship.

As a psychotherapist, you might see ethics codes and laws as constraints—long lists of prohibited behaviors and the punishments involved. However, good work happens when we are working from the lens of "wanting to do the best for the client" (a "positive" principle) rather than from the lens of "this is a hassle, but I don't want to get into trouble" (a "constraint" principle).

Competence: A Basic Ethical Obligation

Because psychotherapy is complex and based on a rich empirical and experiential literature, a basic obligation of therapists is to become and stay competent. Competence is more than good intentions, intuitive understanding, and personal experience. At the same time, competence is not the same as licensure, academic degrees, credentials, attendance at workshops, authored books, and a nice office. Any of these might represent some knowledge and skill level, but they say nothing about ability, diligence, humility, or wisdom.

Psychotherapists do not measure how well they fulfill their obligation to remain competent merely by the absence of harm (Foundation #2); they want clients to receive some level of benefit. From the positive ethics lens, we really want to shoot for the ethical ceiling—we want to do everything on our end of the professional relationship to help the client. We aren't talking perfection here, or working harder than the client. We are talking about keeping track of or monitoring ourselves on five components of competence and assessing where we are on the competence continuum. Kitchener and Anderson (2011) and Welfel (2016) identify four of the five components: knowledge of the literature, skill (technical and clinical) to act on that knowledge, ability (both emotional and physical) to work effectively with the client, and diligence or "going the extra mile" and consistently making sure the client's wellbeing is our top priority. We add a fifth component, which is drawing upon the virtues of humility and wisdom. We need to know when we have hit our limit or boundary of expertise and to recognize that we can't work with every client.

Now you might be thinking, "So, how do I know if and when I am competent? And it sounds like competence or my level of competence can change. Is that right?" Yes, competence can fluctuate—even on a daily basis (Welfel, 2016). To help you assess your own competence, take a look at these questions in each area.

Questions about the knowledge component:

1. What does the current literature say about my clients and their issues?
2. How would I explain my current working knowledge, of theoretical orientations, techniques, etc., to my best clinical supervisor?
3. How do I know the theoretical approach I am using in session is appropriate for my client?

Questions about the skill component:

1. In keeping up with the literature, what new skills am I employing effectively?
2. How do I know that I am implementing these skills effectively?
3. What am I using to assess my effectiveness?

Questions about the ability component:

1. How am I taking care of my own emotional state so that I am able to really be there for my clients?
2. How am I taking care of myself physically so that I am in good health?

Questions about the diligence component:

1. How am I doing with keeping my clients' needs at the top of the priority list?
2. What is my most recent example of "going the extra mile" in my psychotherapy practice?
3. What is currently happening in my practice where I need to go the extra mile?

Questions about the virtue component:

1. How have I used supervision or consultation lately to see if I am staying within my boundaries of expertise?
2. How have I used supervision, consultation, or my own personal therapy lately to assess my current level of effectiveness as a psychotherapist?
3. Is there anything in my current practice that I feel uncomfortable about and wouldn't want it to become known in supervision or consultation?

Multicultural Competence

A critical part of the notion of competence (Foundation #5) concerns our work with people from a variety of cultural backgrounds. Sue et al. (2019) define multicultural competence as having three dimensions: (a) being aware of your own values, beliefs, biases, and notions about humankind and its nature; (b) having a general understanding or knowledge of worldviews different from your own but without negative judgment toward these other worldviews; and (c) having the skills and knowledge to use psychotherapy interventions that are fitting with diverse clients.

We would add a fourth dimension to this list: (d) coming to know your own points of privilege so that you can hear another's experience of being invisible, devalued, disrespected because of their gender, skin color, age, partner choice, economic status, being differently abled, choice of spirituality, and so forth. Having these four dimensions in place would translate into competence to work with individuals different from ourselves. As our world is becoming more and more culturally diverse, it means that multicultural competence is no longer a luxury or add-on of psychotherapists but a foundation of ethical practice.

Now you may be thinking, "Wait a minute! How can I be multiculturally competent in my practice? What if there are some groups that I don't know about? What if there are some worldviews I disagree with? What if …?" These questions are great—they suggest your desire to be transparent. It is easier in the short run to ignore the unfamiliar and avoid areas of disagreement. We are glad you're not doing either of these.

Here is what we say to our students who have asked these questions: First, give yourself some growing room. None of us can be a multicultural expert with all cultures. However, we can be life-long learners and willing to access experience, training, and consultation to gain multicultural competence. Second, not everyone who wants or asks to work with you will be someone you can serve. In this sense, multicultural competence is similar to other types of competence. As a psychotherapist, you will be clear about your limits of competence and it would be unethical for you to go beyond those limits. This is also true about differing worldviews. You may not be able to work competently with someone whose worldview is very different from yours. The issue here should be one of different perspectives without disrespect. Finally, you will probably make better decisions and serve clients well to the extent that sensitivity to, and respect for, diversity is close to your moral core.

Journal Entry: *My Current Location on the Road to Multicultural Competence*

Make a list of three cultures you feel you know a lot about. Write a couple of sentences after each culture explaining how you know about the culture. Then make a list of three cultures you know nothing or very little about, with a couple sentences for each one including a brief statement about your attitudes toward these cultures and a statement of how interested you are in gaining some understanding. (Allow yourself the luxury of being honest.)

Now, on a scale from 1 to 5, with 1 being "not at all descriptive of me" and 5 being "perfectly descriptive of me," rate each of the following thoughts and how much they apply to you at this moment:

_____ I don't need any more information on other cultures than I have now.

_____ I can't work with anybody about whose culture I am not perfectly expert.

_____ I know I have cultural weak spots. I am a little anxious about this but want to develop a strategy to (a) overcome them and/or (b) lessen their impact.

This activity gives you some information about your acculturation journey as it relates to multicultural competence. If you identified with the first statement, you might be adopting a separation strategy. If you identified with the second statement, you might be using an assimilation strategy. If the third statement reflects more of your "current location," you might be using an integration strategy.

Ethical Choice Processes

Having guides for our behavior is one thing, but how do we apply them in real life? Virtually all ethics books include decision-making procedures (Cottone, 2012; Cottone et al., 2007; Knapp et al., 2017). What we have seen is that most models focus on the following steps:

- Identify the problem.
- Develop and analyze alternatives using relevant codes, guidelines, laws, regulations, policies.
- Consult with other professionals.
- Choose, implement, and evaluate the decision.

Many books refer to these models as ethical decision-making models or procedures. Anderson et al. (2006) chose to use the term *ethical choice process* instead. The word *choice* emphasizes the active process of implementing ethical decisions over the purely cognitive exercise of identifying the issues and analyzing relevant codes and principles. The word *process* suggests the fluid, nonlinear, and interactive nature of the model. In some ways it is similar to a feedback loop. New information at any one step can impact the other steps along the way.

As we have seen, making ethical choices involves and is influenced by several factors, including (a) what's in our core—our needs, motivations, and values, (b) the match between our values and those of the profession, (c) our personal character or virtues, (d) moral reasoning, (e) our professional training in ethics, and (f) our professional ethical identity, which has developed through acculturation to the profession. The choice-making process we present here considers these factors and expands on (or augments) the steps above. We have adapted it from a previous work by Anderson et al. (2006).

The centerpiece of the model draws upon Rest's (1984, 1994) four components of moral behavior. Rest developed his model to explain how moral or ethical behavior comes about. He contends that each component has to occur for moral behavior to be the outcome. Although the components are numbered sequentially, Rest states that they don't happen or occur sequentially; rather, they interact with each other. To highlight each of the components and illuminate the process within each one, we present representative questions for therapists to consider. These questions tap into psychotherapists' thinking, motivations, values, needs, and possible conflicts of interest. In addition, the questions show the importance of perspective taking and including client input at appropriate times.

Component 1—Ethical Sensitivity

These questions encourage psychotherapists to develop sensitivity to the issues at hand and how alternative choices will affect others positively and negatively:

- What strikes you as needing some type of response or makes you uncomfortable?
- What is that gut response about?
- What makes you think, "Uh-oh, this doesn't seem right"?
- What makes you think, "Yes, this seems good or right"?
- What are the issues related to diversity and equity? To differences in identities between my client and me? To oppression or discrimination?
- How do my points of privilege affect my sensitivity to this issue?
- If I do something, take some action, how will it impact the interests, wellbeing or expectations/hopes of others?
- How does my value set affect my sensitivity to this issue?
- What new or current values do I need to cultivate?
- What are the possible choices to pursue?
- Who will be affected by the different choices?

Component 2—Formulating an Ethical Plan

These questions prompt psychotherapists to evaluate what they know about the scenario and how various codes, principles, standards, and other guides speak to the ethical problem. They also encourage psychotherapists to view the issue from the client's perspective.

- What do I know about the situation? What are the facts of the case?
- What are the contextual issues?
- What else do I need to know?

- What do ethics codes and other guides have to say about this situation?
- What ethical standards conflict in this situation?
- What are the legal issues involved?
- With whom should I consult? Who would help me see multiple perspectives?
- What do I need to explain or share with the client about the ethical issue?
- If I were the client, what would I hope my psychotherapist would share with me?
- If I were the client, what would I hope my psychotherapist would do?
- Of the different choices I've identified, which one seems to be morally/ethically right, comes closest to the ethical ideal, and reflects the best integration strategies?

Component 3—Ethical Motivation and Competing Values

These questions call for psychotherapists to identify conflicts of interest and their personal motivations and values that are competing with professional values:

- What are my personal motivations and values in this situation?
- What are my professional values and obligations in this situation?
- To what extent is there an overlap and match between the two, and to what extent is there a conflict?
- If I am experiencing acculturation stress, which acculturation strategy am I leaning toward implementing and why?
- To the extent that there is a conflict between my personal values and professional values, what are the options? Can I express my personal values and motivation in a different way? Can I express my professional values and obligations in a different way?
- Do I need to reorganize or reprioritize my personal values? If yes, how?
- Do I need to reorganize or reprioritize my professional values and obligations? If yes, how?
- With whom might I consult to see the conflicts as clearly as possible?
- What core values (personal and professional) are being stretched?
- What core values (personal and professional) are being strengthened?

Component 4—Ethical Follow-Through

These questions prompt implementation of the choice:

- To whom and what (e.g., ethics code, law) must I be accountable? To whom do I want to be accountable?
- Who in my professional circles can encourage or support me to do the right thing?

- What personal and professional values do I need to draw upon to implement my choice?
- What are the possible deterrents for me in following through on what I need to do?
- What did I say in my ethics autobiography that would help me at this point?
- As I implement this choice, what do I need to let the client know?

Tripping Points Along the Way to Ethical Choices

If only it were that easy: Read the ethics codes, be aware of the ethical issues involved in a situation, ask and answer a series of questions, consider alternatives, and choose the right one. Very straightforward, very rational. There's only one fly in this ointment: We are human beings, and human beings are not proficient at rational thinking! Our ethical choice making is influenced by nonrational factors (Knapp et al., 2015; Rogerson et al., 2011) that make it hard to sustain and actualize our professional/ethical identity, stay positive, choose good acculturation strategies—in short, to make good ethical choices in the moment. You may recognize some of these from your introductory, social, or personality psychology courses. You will also notice that these tripping points overlap with each other.

A Compendium of Tripping Points

There is no comprehensive list of tripping points; humans are prone to any number of biases, cognitive tendencies, and influences. Here, we present the tripping points that we have found most useful in helping students and professionals understand some of their difficulty in choice making and acting on those choices. Let's take a situation and move through some variations based on tripping points. Here's the basic situation (adapted from Handelsman, 1998):

> You get a call from a client, Ms. Edwards, who is experiencing significant distress. You know a few things about this client: She is wealthy, she was referred by one of your favorite colleagues who spoke very highly of you, she is experiencing panic attacks, she is very likable and engaging on the phone (she's attractive to you in some way), she wants to make the appointment for tomorrow, and she wants to make the appointment now. You are trying to decide whether you are competent to accept Ms. Edwards as a client.

Ethical Fading

When you first talk to Ms. Edwards, you are thinking about your competence. You are using an ethical frame. If that frame holds, you might decide to refer Ms. Edwards to another therapist because your experience with panic disorders is quite limited. However, as you think about whether to make an appointment, what you want to do may start to overtake what you know you should do (Bazerman et al., 1998; Tenbrunsel & Messick, 2004). You may start thinking about your employer (who may be you!) telling you about the need to increase referrals and billable hours. In other words, you start using a business frame. Or you might use a loyalty/friendship frame: "I can't let my colleague down." Or, "Ms. Edwards is in such pain, it would be cruel to refer her again." Or you might use a convenience frame and make the appointment because you have a session coming up in a few minutes.

Ethical fading may be one reason what people act inconsistently with their moral values (e.g., Batson et al., 1997). As Bazerman and Tenbrunsel (2011) put it, "People have the innate ability to maintain a belief while acting contrary to it" (p. 4).

Anchoring

Anchoring is the tendency people have to pay too much attention to an initial piece of information—which may be irrelevant or arbitrary. That's why salespeople often start their pitches with, "We usually charge $450 for this, but now it's only $325!" In one study, researchers found that physicians diagnosed differently depending on whether they read history or lab test information first—even though the information was the same (Bergus et al., 1998). Your decision about Ms. Edwards might be different depending on whether the initial information you hear is that she suffers from panic attacks or that your favorite colleague referred her. In Chapter 3 we talked about "patient-targeted googling." What if it were called "client-centered digital assessment"? That might change how we see the ethics of the practice.

Bias Blind Spot

We are not good judges of our own biases (Pronin et al., 2002), just as we often find it hard to become aware of our own points of privilege and assess their impact. As you read about each tripping point, you might say to yourself things like, "That wouldn't happen to me; I'm a prudent person and I care too much about clients to let my ethical frame slip." We appreciate your confidence. However, we cannot ignore the possibility that it's *overconfidence*. There are empirical data to show that "individuals overestimate the extent to which they will behave morally in the future" (Sezer et al., 2015, p. 78). We also know about the *Dunning–Kruger Effect*, which states that people with less skill are especially likely to overestimate their skill. Thus, if you were not skilled at treating panic disorders you might be especially prone to overestimating your competence (Dunning, 2011; Epley & Dunning, 2000).

The Substitution Principle

Kahneman (2011) and his colleagues have found that when we are under stress, we may substitute a simple question for a more complex one, and then use the simple answer to substitute for the answer to the complex question. For example, the question, "Am I prepared or trained to provide services to Ms. Edwards?" is a complex one. A simpler question is, "Do I have room in my schedule?" If we answer this question, "Yes," then we may substitute the yes for the answer to the first question. When we think we have a plan or the answer to an ethical question, we may want to take a little time out and think about the question that we have answered, and the questions we haven't.

Another example: You ask yourself, "Am I accepting Ms. Edwards into treatment out of self-interest or for her benefit?" A better question might be: "To what extent is the choice I'm considering consistent with my self-interest, as defined by non-ethical gain as potentially seen by others?" By simplifying the choice into a dichotomy, rather than recognizing that self-interest coexists with benefit to clients, you are losing an opportunity to achieve ethical excellence.

The Availability Heuristic

One of the cognitive shortcuts we take when trying to judge the frequency of some phenomenon is to base that judgment on how easily we recall the phenomenon (Kahneman, 2011). We call upon dramatic, salient, or personal data rather than using a more effortful approach. For example, most people judge dying in accidents to be 300 times more likely than dying from diabetes. In fact, diabetes is 4 times more likely to cause death than accidents (Kahneman, 2011, p. 138). People misjudge the frequencies because accidents are dramatic and covered in the news, whereas diabetes is not. We may judge Ms. Edwards to be a potentially litigious client—and let that skew our choice making—because a colleague told us a story recently about a client with panic disorder who sued his therapist. We may also be more likely to recommend a treatment approach to clients because we use that approach (Grove, 2002), and neglect to recommend treatments that have equal support but that we don't think of quickly.

The Affect Heuristic

Ordinarily, we like to decide what's right and wrong on the basis of values, principles, and other guides. Sometimes, however, we use our affect—positive and negative emotions—instead. Notice that we described Ms. Edwards as *engaging*. We might like her, and our liking may influence our judgment: "She's a nice person, so she will be a good client, which means I can help her." The last two parts of that thought might be true, but notice that they do not follow from the first!

Sometimes we might make decisions that are based too much on negative emotions, which we are especially likely to deny, such as simple dislike or disgust (Pope et al., 2006). Our dislike may be based on something the client has said or done, on their membership in various cultural, religious, or other groups, or simply on our personal background or history.

Loyalty

We may feel loyalty to (in addition to liking) our colleague who referred Ms. Edwards. "I don't want to let him down." We may also feel loyal to our practice partners, employers, family, and others.

Avoidance of Ambivalence and Annoyance

We may rush into a choice that does not reflect our values merely because it is uncomfortable to deal with complex issues, or to deal with them for long. Once again, we may substitute a simple question (e.g., "How do I get this person out of my office?") for a more complex one (e.g., "What is the merit in their complaint against me?"). We can also see this as a "convenience" frame taking over when our ethics frame fades.

Situational Pressures

Sometimes we face situational pressures that, even if they don't deplete our ethical sensitivity, choice making, or values, might make it difficult to carry out our choice. When we're under stress (and many ethical choices are made in stressful situations!), we might be motivated to reduce that stress, quickly, and therefore take shortcuts—in the form of several tripping points. The stress that can influence choice making can be something happening in your life (births, deaths, marriages, divorces, etc.), your career (bills, promotions, etc.), or simply the immediate situation.

Another variable that seems to be a risk factor for ethical lapses is isolation. Sometimes, what we say in our own heads sounds suspiciously like bad reasoning when we say it aloud to somebody else.

Acculturation stress can play a role in our ethical choice making, such as when we need to do some cultural shedding. For example, if your previous employment was in a job where "doing the best you can for everyone" was a core tenet (as in sales, outreach, crisis intervention, etc.), it may simply not feel right to tell Ms. Edwards that you are not a good person to provide services.

Self-Serving Bias

Let's assume, for the sake of argument, that you accepted Ms. Edwards as a client, and her condition worsened. Are you likely to evaluate your behavior as at least partially unethical? No. That's because of a very strong tendency, which psychologists call the *self-serving bias* (Zuckerman, 1979), the tendency to see our own successes as caused by our skills and personalities ("I am a good therapist") and our failures as caused by situational factors ("She was a bad or unmotivated client").

Rationalization

Human beings are so good at generating those reasons when things don't go well that we have a separate name for it: rationalization. Here are some rationalizations that, in our experience, people use, both before and after an unethical behavior (they're all three-word phrases to help you remember; Handelsman, 2017): "Nobody will know." "Just this once." "Everybody does it." "It was convenient!" "Didn't mean to." "Nobody was harmed." "She was crazy."

Confirmation Bias

Once we have made a decision, we have a tendency to look for evidence that our decision was good (ethical), and ignore evidence to the contrary. For example, we might see that Ms. Edwards paid her bills on time and came to therapy for several months—good evidence of her satisfaction with therapy! The fact that she has not improved, or got worse, escapes our attention.

It might be useful to think about how these tripping points happen along the way when we are addressing each of the four components of Rest's model. We might not attend well to the ethical issues involved—compromise our moral/ ethical sensitivity (Component 1)—by virtue of anchoring, a bias blind spot, the availability heuristic, or a self-serving bias. Our moral/ethical reasoning (Component 2) may suffer because we want to avoid ambivalence or annoyance, or because of cognitive tendencies, including anchoring or the substitution principle. We can hijack our own moral/ethical motivation (Component 3) and succumb to competing personal values, motivations, and needs through rationalization, loyalty, and ethical fading. Finally, we can sabotage our moral/ ethical follow-through (Component 4) and not do what we know to be the ethical course by engaging in ethical fading and by not being cognizant enough of the pressures inherent in our situation.

Tripping Points in Action (or, Our Actions at the Tripping Points)

Many instances of unethical behavior result from a "perfect storm" of several tripping points coming together. When tripping points work in concert, their impact on our behavior may be exponential rather than additive. When Ms. Edwards contacts you, you may be new in private practice (isolated and with big rent due on your office), needing good relationships with referring colleagues, in a hurry, enamored with Ms. Edwards, and not in touch with your core. You may find out about her wealth before you hear about her difficulties, and the last client you spoke to just terminated their treatment. Each one of these factors may not have been enough to result in unethical behavior, but the combination *was* enough.

Precursors to Good and Bad Therapist Behaviors: Green and Red Flags

What indicators might there be in our everyday behaviors as therapists that suggest we are navigating our mansion well or tripping on the stairways? In this section we look at good and bad behaviors—behaviors that help us judge whether we are following our professional guides or not, and that indicate potential tripping points or mistakes. We call these behaviors *green flags* and *red flags*.

What Are Green Flags and Red Flags?

When we tell people, "We're writing a book to help psychotherapists stop and really think about their behavioral choices with clients," they often respond with stories of their own experiences with psychotherapists. Here's one story of a therapist who did really good work.

> *I had a friend refer me to his therapist. Man, I was in a world of hurt. Well, I made the call and this therapist was great. I mean it was a safe place for me to share my life story and not feel judged. I remember one time when I really just wanted her to tell me what I should do in a relationship, but she didn't. At the time I felt really frustrated, but as we talked I realized how she was allowing me to take responsibility for myself and not take the easy way out. Looking back, I really like how she helped me figure out what therapy was all about, and what I wanted and needed in a relationship.*

We see this as a great example of ethical work. First, the psychotherapist did a good job of respecting the client's autonomy (Foundation # 3) by encouraging him to arrive at his own answers. Second, our friend says he felt safe and not judged by the therapist. From our view, this therapist was doing good, manifesting beneficence (Foundation #1). We congratulated our friend for finding an ethical psychotherapist who demonstrates some of the green flags we'll share a little later.

On the other hand, we had friends tell us stories about psychotherapists whose behaviors were odd or dubious. Here is one example that demonstrates red flags:

> *You know, I went to a therapist once, and it only lasted one session. I wanted to get over some test anxiety—I learned things well in class, but when I took tests, I couldn't*

do well. So I went to this therapist, and for a lot of the session he talked about things like, oh, getting a lucky pencil—the one I used when I studied and got practice questions right. He said this'd give me confidence. And then, about 45 minutes into the session, he told me I really should stop at a lingerie store on my way home and get a really sexy pair of panties and wear those to the test to make me feel sexy and confident. It kind of creeped me out. I shot out of there and never went back.

Behaviors That Indicate Green Flags

Therapists who are demonstrating ethical or good behaviors are consistently meeting many if not all of the Ethical Foundations. For example, good therapists are humble (Foundation #8), they assume they will have tripping points and try to prevent them, they are in touch with their core, and they are realistic about what they can reasonably expect to accomplish. They are diligent about providing good and clear information to clients so that clients will make better decisions (Foundation #3). Therapists behaving ethically will not guarantee success; however, they will guarantee that they are trying hard to help. Being humble and diligent is also a way of being respectful of clients (Foundation #3). Please note that we used the words "consistently meeting" rather than "perfectly meeting" the Ethical Foundations. None of us is perfect; however, we need to take our responsibility for ethical practice to heart. Kitchener (2000) says it this way:

> Issues of responsibility are some of the most difficult with which to deal in a profession like psychology (counseling) because our work affects other humans. At the same time, we cannot be held to a superhuman standard that never allows for an error in judgment … It is not a standard of perfection. At the same time, we must aspire to provide the most effective services … of which we are capable. (p. 184)

Green flags are indicators that the therapist has good judgment, a good attitude, and a professional approach. The following is a list of some green flags:

- *Amicable Advice About Alternatives.* Therapists will help clients find the best therapy for them, rather than talking them into the therapists' own services.
- *Responsible Referrals.* Therapists will make suggestions about who might be able to provide help for clients, especially when therapy is not working.
- *Informative Information.* Therapists provide useful information about therapy and respond to client questions in understandable language.
- *Clear Consent.* Therapists explicitly seek consent to treatment and revisit this consent at various points in the therapy (for example, when goals change).
- *Cultural Cognizance.* Therapists recognize and seek to understand, within the therapy context, the different identities and worldviews clients hold. Therapists recognize when they are tempted to embrace stereotypes and generalizations and work to steer clear of those.

- *Good Goals.* After the first few sessions (although it could be sooner), therapists and clients need to be clear about therapy goals.
- *Guarded Guarantees.* Therapists are humble and realistic about their work and they do not guarantee success. The only guarantee they do make is to work hard to help.
- *Beneficial Boundary Bolstering.* Therapists will let clients know about boundaries and maintain them as needed for the benefit of the client and their wellbeing.
- *Effective Ethical Explanations.* Therapists will explain the decisions they make.
- *Privilege Perception.* Therapists recognize their points of privilege and how these influence their own behaviors in therapy and sustain systems of oppression for their clients who have been marginalized by society. Therapists address rather than ignore the impacts of racism, sexism, genderism, etc.
- *Common Consultation.* Therapists will avoid professional isolation and tripping points by getting objective opinions from other professionals.
- *Ethical Explorations.* Therapists will ask clients to explore actions and feelings, even when this is uncomfortable. "You're interested in aspects of my private life. I wonder where that might be coming from."
- *Requests for Written Releases.* Therapists request written permission to share information about clients with appropriate professionals, such as physicians or attorneys.
- *Ethical Endings.* Therapists recognize when therapy needs to end (clients have accomplished their goals, or therapy is not being effective), and they facilitate good closure.

Green Flag: Ethical Explanations and Responsible Referrals

Let's return to the scenario with Ms. Edwards: She is pushing you to get her on your calendar for an appointment as early as tomorrow. She is doing her best to be persuasive. You say, "Can you please hold for a few minutes? I'll be right back." You take this time to think: What is my gut response? There's a part of me that says taking Ms. Edwards on as a client doesn't feel right and at the same time I continue to have bills to meet and am flattered that she wants to work with me. Am I competent to help her deal with her panic attacks? I had one course and a workshop but is that enough? I could get supervision, but that's another expense. If I were on an ethics committee, I wouldn't judge one course to be enough! Without the needed competence, I could do more harm than good. Part of my conflict is between my ego being flattered and needing income, but knowing I am currently not competent to work with Ms. Edwards. I can't take her as a client.

You get back on the line with Ms. Edwards, "Thank you for waiting, and for your interest in working with me. I feel honored. However, I do not have the necessary experience and training to do good work around panic attacks. But what I can do to help is to give you the names of three other therapists. I know each of them professionally and they have experience working with clients like you who are dealing with panic attacks. I know this is not the answer you were hoping for. I understand that. But I want you to work with someone who has sound experience in this area and is better equipped to help you."

Questions:

How does this response strike you? What might you think about or say differently?

If you put yourself in Ms. Edwards' shoes, how might you take this response?

GREEN

Behaviors That Indicate Red Flags

Remember the story about a therapist suggesting that our friend buy and wear a "sexy pair of panties" to boost her confidence for taking a test? During this conversation with our friend, we talked about the fact that this suggestion might have been an innocent comment and not a sexual overture. Dealing with sex in therapy is just like dealing with money, marriage, anxiety, depression, and other aspects of human existence. However, we also said that making this particular comment, innocent or not, showed extremely poor judgment by the therapist. We thought our friend was smart to leave that office and not go back. If the psychotherapist was not a sexual pervert, he may have been showing a preview (aka a red flag) of more bad choices to come.

Sexual remarks made out of context, or undue focus on sex, is one of the easiest precursors or red flags to spot. But there are lots of other warning signs that are smaller, more subtle, and harder to detect. At a minimum, red flags are indicators of poor judgment and/or a lack of ethical sensitivity and training. They are certainly signs that therapists may not be taking their professional responsibilities as seriously as they should. We are not saying that each of these red flags is, in itself, unethical or unprofessional behavior. We are saying, however, that the red flags may at least be precursors to more serious problems. The following is a list of red flags:

- *Everybody's Everything.* Therapists convey, directly or indirectly, that they can handle every problem, often because of what good therapists they are. This shows a naïve and simplistic attitude toward complex phenomena (human emotion and behavior). This red flag could also be called Lacking Clarity on the Limits of Competence.

- *Overlooked Oppression.* Therapists shy away from recognizing overt or covert collision with systems of oppression. They may invalidate the discriminatory experiences of clients whose identities are marginalized in society. Their response is often one of disbelief, minimization, or rationalization.

- *Dissing the Different.* Therapists are overly disparaging of other therapists or other approaches. Related red flags might be: *Excessive Enthusiasm for Exclusive Enterprises*, in which therapists will try to sell one type of therapy, or one answer to all problems, rather than appreciating that there are lots of ways to solve problems. For example, "What you need is hypnosis! It works wonders for all my clients, and for me." *Defensive Declarations*, in which therapists will "pull rank" when challenged, rather than address clients' concerns. For example, "You're not supposed to ask me that question. I'm the therapist here."

- *Logistical Laxity.* This refers to evidence of sloppiness. Forgetting appointments, not having the right forms available, not keeping adequate records—all indicate that for some reason therapists are not taking care of business.

- *Exciting Exceptions Equal Excruciating Effects.* Therapists make exceptions to their usual policies. They might say something like: "I wouldn't do this with my other clients, but ..." One such exception may be a red flag of *Shared Secrets*: Therapists are secretive about certain activities in therapy. "This'll be just our little secret."

- *Compromised Confidentiality and Porous Privacy.* Therapists will violate client privacy and confidentiality by sharing information about them with others. For example, therapists leave paperwork and correspondence on the desk or on the computer monitor with clients' names within the field of vision of anyone who might come into their office. Therapists may also share information about one client with another client. The most problematic example is a full disclosure, with names and/or other identifying information about some experience of clients. This conduct can also take the form of bragging, with therapists telling stories about their triumphs. Porous privacy can be quite subtle, however, like simply illustrating a point with an example with too much detail. We'll spend time on these issues in Chapter 6.

- *Bad Boundaries.* We devote Chapter 5 to boundary issues. For now, here is a sample of boundary-related behaviors to watch out for:

  - *Intimations of Inappropriate Intimacy.* Therapists blur boundaries between a professional and personal relationship, resulting in harm to the client.
  - *Invidious Invitations.* Therapists invite clients to functions or events that are not part of therapy.

- **Reprehensible Rationalizations.** Therapists offer explanations to clients for behaving unethically that may sound good but are only rationalizations for breaking the rules. The simplest and perhaps most dangerous: "Just this once." Other tripping points may be evident in related red flags of *Cognitive Contortions* or *Encroaching Emotions*.
- **Spiritual Selling.** Discussing spiritual or religious issues in therapy may be just fine if it is related to clients' goals. But it is *not* a good sign when therapists force their spiritual perspective on clients or invite clients to their place of worship.
- **Sideline Solicitations.** Therapists offer a service or product for sale that is not part of therapy. For example, they offer to do clients' taxes, or to sell clients their old phone or notebook.
- **Counterproductive Curiosity About Clients.** Therapy, by its very nature, deals with very personal experiences and issues. When therapists get too interested in hearing personal details that are not therapeutically relevant, they are letting their own interests (prurient or otherwise) get in the way.

We anticipate at least two possible reactions from you as you read through the list of red flags and the red flag stories throughout the rest of the book. Your first reaction might be, "No therapist would do anything that extreme/insensitive/stupid/ unethical." Some of these examples are more extreme than others, but we want you to know that they are all based on actual cases we are familiar with—although we've disguised identities and facts to preserve privacy.

The second reaction you might have is, "*I* would never do anything like that!" We encourage you to bear in mind that good people can and do end up doing unethical things, often unintentionally (Bazerman & Tenbrunsel, 2011). And remember the bias blind spot: We are human, with complex motivations, and psychotherapy is a complex, unique, powerful, and fragile process. Consequently, we are all capable of unethical behaviors. You will get more out of these stories by considering the red flags and tripping points as possible conditions under which you could act similarly, rather than creating distance between you and the therapists depicted.

Red Flag: Logistical Laxity

Consider the following story:

Sarah paced up and down the long, thin hallway in the office building. Dr. Horne's office was at the far end of the hallway, away from the elevators, so Sarah would not miss spotting Dr. Horne. It was already 8:25, and they had an 8:00

appointment. Sarah was happy that Dr. Horne made this early appointment (rather than the usual 8:30) so she could make it to a work meeting on time, but now she felt like there might not be any session at all.

At the stroke of 8:30, Dr. Horne came rushing out of the elevator, her face hardly visible behind a large purse, a leather briefcase, a laptop case, several paperback books, and a tote bag from the local public radio station. Even while carrying all that, Dr. Horne was jiggling her keyring loudly, trying to lay her finger on her office keys. "Good morning!" she said brightly.

Sarah said, "Uh, we were scheduled for 8:00."

"Oh, were we? I must have forgotten to check my book. Don't we usually meet at 8:30?"

"Yes, but we changed it last time, remember?"

"Oh yes," Dr. Horne responded. "But we can go a few minutes later. My next client won't mind."

That's really not the point, thought Sarah. She felt let down when she thought Dr. Horne wasn't going to show at all. And besides, she was wanting to do some heavy work. Now it was hard for her to "gear up" again to have a good session. Should she just leave? Would Dr. Horne charge her?

Here are some questions to consider:

- What's it like to be "stood up" in this way? How does it make you feel?
- Which of the Ethical Foundations might Dr. Horne have violated?
- How serious would you judge the violations to be? For example, how much harm was done?
- Suppose Sarah is from a marginalized group and Dr. Horne is White and has multiple points of privilege. What are the additional issues of concern here?
- What virtues might Dr. Horne need to cultivate?
- How often are you late for appointments?
- What other behaviors might you exhibit that would be included in "logistical laxity"? Sloppy record-keeping? Forgetfulness? How do they influence the relationships you are in? How might they influence your therapy relationships? What acculturation strategies might be reflected in logistical laxity? What strategies might be good alternatives?

Ethics Autobiography, Part 2

In Chapter 2 you started your ethics autobiography by discussing your ethics of origin, your core. In this part of the Ethics Autobiography, we ask you to explore your professional culture.

If you are a student or a new professional, we encourage you to start here with these questions. If you are a practicing psychotherapist, you can focus on your initial training as you answer these questions, or you can skip to the next set of questions.

- What have you learned about the culture of psychotherapy that you did not expect?
- What have you learned about or been asked to do that has been counterintuitive, surprising, or puzzling?

This will get you started focusing on your acculturation tasks. If you find a lot that has been counterintuitive you may be facing acculturation stress or crises—large disconnects between your goals/needs/motivations/values and your ability to meet those goals as a psychotherapist.

Here are some other questions to consider:

- Which parts of your new profession fit easily into who you are at your core and which parts do not (did not) seem like such a good fit?
- How have your personal relationships changed as a result of becoming a psychotherapist?
- If you have been in the profession long enough, take a few minutes to answer these questions:
  - How has the profession changed since you entered it?
  - How have you changed since you first became a therapist?
  - What tripping points have you noticed?
  - As you look back, what aspects of your professional development may have been an interaction between your personal changes and changes in the profession?
- One final question: What personal and professional changes might you need to deal with in the next few years (e.g., divorce, retirement, empirically supported treatments, the rise of coaching)?

Conclusion

In Part I we invited you to explore your core and become aware of who you are, your needs, motivations, values, virtues. These are the foundation of your professional ethical identity. We also invited you to consider your points of privilege and the social responsibility you have as a professional. We followed this discussion with exploring ethical acculturation—developing your professional/ethical identity. In this chapter we presented, in broad terms, the principles and values that characterize the profession of psychotherapy and an ethical choice-making process. Thus, the basic foundations of acculturation are now in place.

Now it is time to explore (or re-explore) the culture of psychotherapy in enough detail to give you a sense of how your acculturation is progressing. In Part II we go more deeply into the ethical traditions and themes of psychotherapy, including boundaries, confidentiality, informed consent, supervision, and termination. As you work through these chapters, please refer back to the journal entries and exercises you have done thus far. Maintaining your awareness of your own core (needs, motivations, values, backgrounds), along with the Ethical Foundations of Psychotherapy, will help you avoid moving too far into the strategies of assimilation, separation, or marginalization, and will keep your eyes on *your own* path toward excellence and a healthy and vibrant professional/ethical identity.

Part II

The Nuts and Bolts of Psychotherapy Ethics

5

Boundaries and Multiple Relationships in the Psychotherapy Relationship

Thus far in our time in the mansion—walking up the spiral staircase and visiting some of the rooms, you've explored your core—your moral self; you've looked at your points of privilege and their relationship to oppression and discrimination; you've started building your professional ethical identity; you've gained some understanding of the professional culture and what it looks like to become part of the culture. Now we are ready to explore parts of the mansion more specifically. We start these explorations with boundaries and multiple relationships. Before we get into definitions and discussions, please read through and reflect on the following scenarios.

Food for Thought: *Boundaries*

We present five scenarios for your consideration:

Greta was horribly distraught. She had been telling Mr. Desmond for the last 40 minutes about the argument she just had with her mom. Mr. Desmond noticed that their time was coming to a close. When he mentioned they had 10 minutes left, Greta went into more tears and sounded even more emotional than before. This was a pattern, Mr. Desmond noticed. As the sessions were starting to end, Greta seemed to get more emotional and animated, and sometimes even begged Dr. Desmond for a couple of extra minutes. Sometimes Mr. Desmond would let the session exceed the 50 minutes by 3 to 8 minutes. On other occasions when Mr. Desmond had another appointment, he would actually open the door and have to wave Greta out the door—confirming next week's appointment as they walked down the hall.

Don was excited to share the news with Dr. Woods. He got a promotion at work and felt like Dr. Woods had been a big part of this positive outcome. Because of Dr. Woods and the good work they'd done, Don was more confident and really believed there wasn't anything he couldn't accomplish if he set his mind to it. Don couldn't thank Dr. Woods enough. At the end of a session, Don slipped an envelope onto

Dr. Woods's desk. Before leaving for the day, Dr. Woods saw the envelope and opened it to find a thank you card and gift card for the most expensive restaurant in town.

Winston had been seeing Dr. Konitz weekly over the last two months. His initial concerns were about his work environment, but the topic had shifted to personal relationships. In this session, Dr. Konitz sensed Winston's attention was distracted. He appeared to be interested in something on her desk. He would gaze briefly in that direction, squint just a little, and then quickly refocus back to her. After the fifth time, Dr. Konitz stopped mid-sentence and asked, "Winston, I notice you keep looking over at my desk and trying to focus on something of interest over there." Winston sat up straight in his chair and said, "Well, I'm just curious. Who's the person in the picture with you? I don't think it's your husband because I haven't seen you wear a wedding ring or, you know, stuff like that." Dr. Konitz was taken by surprise. She responded with, "That's my late husband—he died of alcoholism 4 years ago."

Dr. Coleman had just discussed her finances with an accountant, who talked about some necessary changes to make in her finance plans. Dr. Coleman didn't know much about financial planning and felt lost. She remembered that one of her former clients, Sophie, was a financial planner with a big company. She had talked about her promotion due to her success with several portfolios, and about the overall success of the company. Dr. Coleman looked up Sophie's company on the internet. While she was at it, she also looked up Sophie's LinkedIn profile and Facebook account, curious about Sophie's professional and personal successes. The next day Dr. Coleman called Sophie's s company to get an appointment with a financial planner. The receptionist got Dr. Coleman scheduled with the first person available, which was in two weeks. Dr. Coleman felt hopeful. Later that day, Dr. Coleman got an email confirming her appointment with Ms. S. Brown. Dr. Coleman put the appointment in her calendar, feeling she had made a good next step. A few minutes later, she remembered that Brown was Sophie's last name. She shrugged her shoulder and thought, "It will probably be ok. What's the chances that Sophie will need more therapy in the future?"

Anita has been seeing her therapist, Dr. Bolden, for several months. Toward the end of a recent session, Dr. Bolden begins sharing little tidbits about his own relationships. His wife, he tells Anita, is frequently out of town. He goes on to say that their interests, which were similar at one time, are now very different. He hints about their sex life being almost nonexistent. Anita feels a little funny about what Dr. Bolden is saying, but rationalizes it as an issue of trust in their therapeutic relationship. She even feels a little honored by his confiding in her. A couple of sessions later, Dr. Bolden compliments Anita on the progress she's made as he literally pats her on the back. This makes Anita feel really good. As he continues to keep his hand on Anita's shoulder, Dr. Bolden suggests that, as a kind of celebration, they meet for their next session at a quaint little restaurant near the office. Feeling only a little uncomfortable about the dinner but very pleased with praise by a therapist, Anita accepts the invitation. At the restaurant, Dr. Bolden makes a sexual advance, which

Anita angrily rebuffs. After only a few more sessions, Anita's condition worsens and she quits therapy.

Given what we have discussed thus far, and the discussions you may already have had in class, what are your concerns about the above scenarios? What red flags do you see, if any, and when do the red flags become apparent? What tripping points might there be for each of our therapists? When does your moral core say, "Oh no, that's problematic." At what point or points in the scenarios do you see the psychotherapists' behaviors no longer appropriate to their role? What are some possible therapist needs and motivations being played out? What ethical foundations might they be violating? What virtues might they not have enough, or too much, of? What might you speculate about what acculturation strategies they are using?

Because psychotherapy occurs behind closed doors, with usually only the client and therapist in the room, misconceptions about what should and should not be part of the relationship abound. Movies, internet programming, and novels routinely portray therapists and clients interacting in ways that go beyond the therapy relationship—for example, therapists having romantic encounters with clients or adopting a client to be their child. In addition, family members or friends might mention that they had a therapy session at a coffee shop, or that their therapists talked a lot about their own troubles during sessions. These examples suggest the therapist is engaged in behaviors that go beyond the therapist role; they go beyond the boundaries of the therapy relationship.

Boundaries: What They Are and Why They Are So Important

We can think of boundaries in two ways. First, there are boundaries between therapists and clients. Second, there are boundaries around the role(s) that therapists play, differentiating those behaviors that are part of the role of therapist and those that are not (Gutheil & Gabbard, 1993).

When therapists get too close to their clients, when they engage in behaviors that are not part of therapy, or when they play roles other than "therapist"—such as "business partner" or "lover," -the therapists' obligations and the clients' expectations shift so much that the risk of harm goes way up. You can think of boundary violations as therapists and clients moving outside the mansion or to rooms where they don't belong. The stairways—the choice process regarding boundaries—can sometimes be ill-lit and treacherous. Tripping points abound. There are situations where psychotherapists find it hard to discern correct choices and they need to consider aspects of other roles, such as when they serve clients of color or clients with minoritized identities (see Chapter 2).

Boundaries in the therapy relationship provide safety and protection for the clients from being used by therapists for their personal gratification (Simon, 1992). They provide the necessary space for therapists' objectivity and clients' sense of safety. Because clients are vulnerable when they share personal information, they need to trust that their therapist is in the relationship primarily for the client's benefit (Welfel, 2016). Thus, boundaries provide a framework which allows therapy to work by delineating role obligations and expectations for both therapists and clients (Kitchener & Anderson, 2011; Smith & Fitzpatrick, 1995).

When considering the cases that began the chapter, you can look at what the therapists did and ask: "Is this what a therapist does?" (Gutheil & Gabbard, 1993, p. 190). Are the therapists' behaviors appropriate for the role of therapist? You can also look at whether the therapists are getting too emotionally close to their clients, and whether they have clients' needs at the forefront of their choice making.

Discussions about boundaries have been evolving over the past four decades. The main foundations of beneficence, nonmaleficence, justice, and respect for client autonomy are paramount. Blurring boundaries makes it easier and more likely to exploit clients by abusing our power in our role as a psychotherapist (Birchmore, 2015, p. 1). However, the prevailing wisdom has evolved from rigid parameters—"Just don't do it!"—to a more thoughtful and nuanced approach: "The decisions can be complex; we need to think clearly about why and how boundaries might need to be articulated and actualized in various situations."

More and more, authors have been recognizing practice context and cultural considerations regarding boundaries (e.g., Barnett, 2007; Lazarus, 2007; Speight, 2012; Sue et al., 2019; Vasquez, 2007). As Vasquez (2007) suggests, "The more frequent challenge for most psychotherapists is whether or not to rigidly apply boundaries or allow for 'permeable' boundaries that one crosses from time to time. One of the risks in misapplying unnecessary boundaries for culturally different individuals is that of re-creating shaming, oppressive experiences for racially and ethnically diverse clients, most of whom may have histories of discriminatory, shaming, and oppressive experiences" (p. 407).

In other parts of life, the boundaries between ourselves and others, and role boundaries we have in our relationships with other people, are often fluid. Where one relationship ends and the other begins is not always clear—nor does it always need to be. For example, we buy insurance from our friends, we invite our neighbors to come with us to community events, and we play cards or have barbecues with the parents of our children's friends. In addition, boundaries within some relationships are in flux. For example, as a child moves into adulthood, the boundaries between the child and parents change. Another change occurs with boundaries and roles when adult children move into a care-giving role with their aging parents.

The therapeutic relationship, however, is fragile—therefore, we need to be more aware and think more intentionally about boundaries. We need to be aware that we can cross boundaries because of many factors, including our unmet personal needs, unexamined or mixed motives, lack of contact with our core, and a lack of self-care.

These factors, along with situational pressures and an array of cognitive and emotional tripping points, can increase the likelihood of being insensitive, distracted, or self-serving.

Because of the fragility of the therapy relationship and the potential for the abuse of power, therapists have a "fiduciary duty" toward clients (Jorgenson et al., 1997, p. 49). According to Jorgenson et al., "a fiduciary relationship exists when one party, the fiduciary, accepts the trust and confidence of another party, the entrustor, and agrees to act only in the entrustor's best interest" (p. 51). By entering into the therapy relationship, we accept the trust and confidence the client places in us, and in our competence to act in ways that are in their best interests. We understand that we have the power to "exert undue influence" (p. 51) upon clients; maintaining good, clear, healthy boundaries helps us use our power for optimal therapeutic benefit. Changes in boundaries can compromise the goals and focus of the professional relationship.

In other words, it is the line between the therapy relationship and some other type of relationship with the client. Let's take a look at another scenario.

Red Flags: *Invidious Invitations and Reprehensible Rationalizations*

> Right as they are getting ready to start their session, Dr. Vaughan hears her stomach growl. She stands up, looks at Lena and says, "Look, I missed my lunch and my stomach is talking to me. Maybe you're hungry too? How about if we walk down to the coffee shop on the corner, find a quiet place there and do our session while eating?" Lena knows this isn't a recognized part of therapy … but she IS hungry! And Dr. Vaughan is making a good case for lunch being very convenient.

In reflecting on this story, think through the following questions:

- What are your concerns with Dr. Vaughan's suggestion?
- If you are the client, Lena, what are you feeling besides being hungry? What do you think of the suggestion?
- Based on your initial reaction, what or how would you respond to Dr. Vaughan's suggestion?
- Put yourself in Dr. Vaughan's position. Besides being hungry and wanting to get lunch, what are other possible needs and motivations behind your request or suggestion? As a way to explore issues of justice and the affect heuristic, ask yourself this question: Might you have given any of your clients the same invitation, or is there something you like about Lena that allowed you to make this exception?

- Think about Dr. Vaughan's fiduciary responsibility. On a scale from 1 to 10, 1 being "not upholding her duty at all" and 10 being "perfectly trustworthy," where would you rank her behavior, and why?
- What acculturation strategy might be reflected in Dr. Vaughan's behavior? What behaviors would you encourage her to consider as she works toward integration?
- What if Dr. Vaughan suggested a session at another location? A nearby park? In her vehicle? In her home?

Boundary Extensions, Boundary Crossings, and Boundary Violations

As we stated earlier, boundaries exist to protect clients from therapists' self-interest and exploitation, and to facilitate client autonomy and benefit. Now, let's drill a little deeper into three types of boundary alterations: extensions, crossings, and violations.

A boundary *extension* is a slight and temporary modification of the boundary that would likely benefit the client; the roles of both the therapist and the client remain in place. For example, a client begins to talk about a very difficult issue toward the end of a session and clearly becomes upset. A therapist might let the 50 minutes move into 55 or 59 minutes to give the client some time to reset their emotions before they leave. Of course, if this became a pattern, as it seemed to be with Greta, then the boundary extension is probably not helpful; the therapist needs to address the pattern. Another boundary extension might be when a client sees his or her therapist outside of the therapeutic context and blurts out the need to talk about a situation the next time they meet. Rather than shut the client totally down at the moment, the therapist gently reassures the client they will discuss the issue first thing next session and tries to move the conversation to another issue.

A boundary *crossing* is a departure "from commonly accepted clinical practice that may or may not benefit the client" (Smith & Fitzpatrick, 1995, p. 500). There is temporary change in the relationship—a suspension of roles by both the therapist and the client (Barnett, 2015; Kitchener & Anderson, 2011) meant to benefit the client. The intention may be to benefit the client, but this suspension of roles, a departure from the usual way of doing clinical practice, needs to be identified and discussed between the therapist and client. For example, a client invites his therapist to his wedding and the reception that follows. If the therapist decides to go because it might be of benefit to the client, the therapist's role in that setting is a guest—albeit with some professional parameters still in place (e.g., the client's confidentiality is honored). The therapist and client obviously need to discuss the situation in the therapy, before and after the event or situation, to correct any missteps that occurred, reduce the risk of complications in the relationship, and to maximize whatever benefit might come out of the boundary crossing. In some cultures, clients may expect psychotherapists in the community to participate in weddings, memorial services, and other events to support them and the community.

Another example of a possible boundary crossing is when a client gives a therapist a gift, as Don did with Dr. Woods. In this case, Dr. Woods didn't find out about the gift until opening the envelope. Dr. Woods asks himself whether Don will benefit, and may not be able to answer this question without pursuing a conversation with Don. Dr. Woods will consider a range of factors, such as the cultural context of the gift.

Boundary *violations* are serious breaches that are potentially harmful to the therapeutic relationship and exploitative of clients (Gutheil & Gabbard, 1993). They are clear departures from generally accepted standards of practice (Welfel, 2016). As Martinez (2000) says, "with significant harm and exploitation, the crossing is then labeled a violation" (p. 45) Here are some examples:

- engaging in sexual behavior with a client;
- financially exploiting a client;
- inviting a client to join you at your place of worship or a spiritual retreat;
- asking for more information about situations than is necessary.

All these boundary violations are disrespectful to clients (Foundation #3). They negate the trust therapists and clients are trying to build. They will likely cause harm (Foundation #2), make clients feel emotionally and psychologically confused, and take the focus off of clients' goals.

The last bullet, "asking for more information about situations than is necessary," can be one of the trickiest to assess in the moment. Our role is to ask questions that encourage clients to share information about themselves, yet at times our personal curiosity may take over. Here is an important place to tune into our motivations.

Another element to consider is whether the therapist is making an exception to a professional or ethical policy. The thinking on the therapist's side is, "Just this once might be ok." Or "I think this could benefit the client even though it's not the usual practice." Now is the time for that therapist to stop and remember the *Exciting Exceptions* and *Bad Boundaries* red flags, including *Reprehensible Rationalizations*. The therapist might also recognize some tripping points—if they want to avoid the bias blind spot! For example, the therapist's ethical frame may be fading, perhaps because of the affect heuristic.

The current literature on boundaries reflects a continuum of perspectives regarding what is right, or beneficial, and what is wrong, or harmful. We consider the continuum, and the resulting debates in the literature, as a good thing. Of course, there are some boundaries that all ethical psychotherapists would say are clearly violations and should never be crossed because the risk of harm is so great (Gabbard,

1989). However, many other decisions about boundaries are complex, and therapists need to think well about a variety of factors.

Among the elements of the therapy relationship that influence our deliberations are setting, culture, race, class, and the specific, unique composition of the therapeutic relationship of the individuals in the therapy room (Brown, 1994; Speight, 2012). Gutheil and Gabbard (1993) discuss multiple factors that reflect boundaries, including roles, place or space, self-disclosure, time, gifts, language, physical touch, and clothing.

Sometimes therapists alter boundaries out of "good intentions." Dr. Vaughan, in our last example, might have genuinely believed that she was maximizing her time and potential for a good therapy outcome by conducting therapy while eating, albeit in a secluded part of a restaurant. However, intentions are complex and hard to gauge from the outside. As we said in Chapter 1, others do not always understand or experience the therapist's intensions as virtuous. It is hard to see Dr. Vaughan's good intentions because her behavior is also consistent with selfish intentions. What can be seen, and what ethics committees, state licensing boards, and others use to make their judgments of the ethics of actions, is more often (a) the effects, rather than the intentions, of the actions, and (b) whether the behaviors themselves constitute unethical behavior—whether they line up or don't line up with the role of therapist.

There is some evidence for the *slippery slope* model of boundary violations—that small boundary extensions or crossings lead to violations (Gabbard & Lester, 2003). The slippery slope model would suggest that therapists avoid all behaviors that might extend or cross a boundary, no matter how small. However, some authors suggest that a more nuanced approach might be more useful (Martinez, 2000), and that therapists' fear of the slippery slope can hinder genuine, real connection between therapist and client (Lazarus, 2007; Speight, 2012; Zur & Lazarus, 2002). We agree that the slope may not be as slippery as it seems—not all boundary extensions or crossings lead to violations. However, the slippery slope visual is a good reminder that boundary decisions are fraught with tripping points and must be considered intentionally. For example, Dr. Vaughan may have been feeling stressed that particular day, and in addition to liking Lena, she may have been engaging in a self-serving bias. "I am offering this boundary extension because I'm a good therapist, not because I'm hungry." Her evaluation of Lena's acceptance of the lunch invitation might be an example of a confirmation bias: "This behavior was not harmful to Lena because she went to lunch with me."

In the literature, boundary extensions are usually grouped together with boundary crossings; however, we find it useful to think of extensions and crossings as distinct. Again, a boundary extension is meant to benefit the client and both roles remain intact. Referring to the slippery slope model, the therapist is willing to adjust but not remove the boundary of the professional relationship to benefit the client for a specific situation. However, remember that the intent of an action does always equal the impact. Thus, the therapist remains aware of how this adjustment is affecting the relationship, often by discussing the extension with the client.

In terms of the slippery slope, the extension is located just *before* there is a downturn or slope. A crossing, a temporary suspension of roles by both the therapist and the client intended for good, occurs further along, after the downturn but not too far down. For us, boundary violations are too far down, perhaps toward the bottom of the slope. At the time the boundary is violated, the client might not recognize they have experienced harm. That realization can come later. Here are a couple of red flag stories with which to practice. As you read them, ask yourself what is in the story, or would need to be there, to judge the behaviors as extensions, crossings, or violations.

Red Flag: *Counterproductive Curiosity About Clients*

When they were going over a traumatic event from her childhood, Ella understood that it was helpful to tell her story fully to her therapist, Dr. Hunter. Now, however, no matter what topic Ella is discussing, Dr. Hunter sits forward in her chair and asks for explicit details. Ella thinks, "Why is my therapist so interested in names, dates, locations, and sexual positions!"

Red Flags: *Spiritual Selling, Invidious Invitations, and Shared Secrets Seem Suspicious*

Dr. Pinkus has been seeing Anna for stress management for several weeks. At the end of one session, Anna wishes Dr. Pinkus a happy Easter. "Where are you worshipping Easter?" asks Dr. Pinkus.

"Oh, my husband and I don't belong to a church," replies Anna. As she says this she sees what can only be described as a dark cloud drift over Dr. Pinkus's face.

"What a shame!" exclaims Dr. Pinkus. "We would love to have you come to our church!"

Anna is taken aback. She has never raised the subject of religion during the therapy, and was only wishing Dr. Pinkus a happy Easter just to be polite. This invitation seems too quick, too removed from therapy, and a little creepy. After all, Anna thinks, who is this "we" that she's talking about? Does she invite all her clients to her church? Does she tell her family or friends at her church that she invites clients to worship with them? "No thanks," she manages to say.

Dr. Pinkus says, "I think it's important to have a church to go to. If you came to mine, we wouldn't have to tell anybody I'm your therapist. In fact, if any-body asks, it would be better if we just say that we're friends. Or, how about we pretend to be strangers and that you found the church in the phone book."

Anna now feels herself getting angry. This isn't the kind of honesty that Dr. Pinkus has been encouraging Anna to develop!

Red Flag: *Exciting Exceptions Equal Excruciating Effects*

Jeanne, who had been laid off from her office manager job at age 52, gets the name of a "cute" therapist from a friend of hers who met him when she took skiing lessons from him last winter. The therapist, Dr. Parker, prides himself on being able to relate especially well to women who are suffering from loneliness and depression. He tells Jeanne that she doesn't have to call him Doctor, and, interest-ingly enough, he never really tells her what his doctorate is in or where it's from.

During the second session, Jeanne is discussing her financial problems when Dr. Parker interrupts her to say, "Listen, I know I shouldn't do this, but how would you like to be my secretary for just a few weeks? I'm writing a book and could use some extra help."

Jeanne has never been in therapy, but she has this funny feeling inside and asks tentatively, "Is that ok, I mean, hiring a client of yours?"

"Well technically," Dr. Parker says, "it's not really considered a good thing. But we're both mature people, and I'm sure we can handle the issues that may come up." Even as she struggles not to, Jeanne finds herself feeling flattered and special. And spending "extra" time with Dr. Parker might help her feel less lonely.

Think about the motivations of the therapists in these red flag stories. How do you see the boundaries being addressed? By their actions, are the therapists bolstering or maintaining boundaries, or are they extending, crossing, or vio-lating boundaries? What tripping points might they not be seeing? How would you encourage each therapist to move toward an integration strategy? What virtues might they need to develop, bolster, or reorganize?

Common Boundary Issues

Let's take a look at some common boundary issues in more detail.

Giving Advice

How do you know when you are giving too much advice, the wrong kind of advice, or when you should not even be giving advice at all? Giving advice is a very controversial issue and therapists' practices vary widely, based on their theoretical orientation, clients' culture, and practice context.

Food for Thought: *Acculturating to Giving Advice*

Think of your own culture and how advice is valued or used in relationships. Think also about your family of origin, friendships, previous job situations, and so forth.

- How much specific advice do you generally give in these relationships?
- What role does advice play in these relationships?
- What kinds of advice do you find most and least helpful?
- To what extent might you give advice as a way of minimizing ambivalence and annoyance?
- Do you sometimes give advice on a simple question as a way of avoiding a more complex question?
- What types of acculturation strategies might you be tempted to use regarding giving advice when it comes to working with your clients?
- For experienced therapists: How has your experience of sharing advice changed? Why might that be?
- For both the novice and veteran therapist, how might you think about moving toward integration?

Depending on the context of your work and the client's culture, an early red flag might be that you are giving too much advice, especially early in therapy. In this case, it becomes apparent to you and probably to the client that you are there to "fix" them or their situation. At the same time, some clients of color, because of their culture, will expect that you are an expert and have some wisdom to share about their situation.

How do you know what course of action to choose to honor the appropriate boundary? First, it is important to know how your client identifies culturally. The answer to this question can give you some initial sense of what "advice giving" might mean to them. Next, it is important to explore their expectations of you as the expert in the room. The third step is to clarify the nature and meaning of advice. Here we can differentiate between we call *process advice* and *substantive advice*. Process advice consists of suggestions for how to go about solving problems, or how to make the most of therapy. Substantive advice consists of suggestions for specific solutions to the problems. The key here is that we want to honor our client's identities, honor their right to autonomous choice making (Foundation #3), and be congruent with our theoretical approach. Ultimately, we want to be clear about our needs, motivation, and values in the process and strive to use integration strategies.

As we alluded to in the Food for Thought, giving advice can sometimes be influenced by our tripping points. Our ethical frame, including respect for autonomy, may fade in comparison to frames dealing with convenience or our need to be seen as wise or knowledgeable. Attempting to solve a client's immediate problem may mask more complex issues that need more attention. And we may use the confirmation bias when we find instances of our advice to clients having worked.

Therapist Self-Disclosure

Therapist self-disclosure can arise in various ways. We may feel that sharing a personal story about an issue might help clients. Or clients may ask us personal questions, as in the case of Winston and Dr. Konitz earlier. It is natural for our clients to want to know about us as people (Braaten & Handelsman, 1997; Braaten et al, 1993). It can even feel good, perhaps flattering, to have a client curious about who we are. Handling self-disclosure is an issue of our core—our needs, motivations, and values all play roles in our decisions about when and how much to disclose. Self-disclosure is a key acculturation task, because decisions vary so much depending on whether the context is personal or professional and whether it will derail the focus of the session or further the therapeutic relationship.

Indeed, research has suggested that self-disclosure can have positive impact on the therapy process (Myers & Hayes, 2006). Thus, some types and amounts of disclosure can be justified by the principle of beneficence. Clients of color and other marginalized clients may see therapist visibility as a necessary part of building rapport and a good working relationship. Information is a source of power in a relationship. As Vasquez (2007) suggests, marginalized clients may experience a therapist's self-disclosure as an avenue of "mutuality and connection" and sense of "more power in the relationship" (p. 407).

Arguments in favor of self-disclosure also revolve around the virtues of honesty and openness. Psychotherapy, like other intimate relationships, values transparency, honesty, and disclosure. Therefore, some personal questions from clients are understandable, appropriate, and might be important to answer.

If a client asks you about children and being in a marriage or significant relationship, they may be appropriately trying to get a handle on your "practical" experience of their issues. It might be appropriate and helpful to respond, "Yes, I have two children," or "Yes, I am married," and leave it at that. But even here, you need to be careful to bolster the boundary by not answering with too much personal information. Dr. Konitz responded to Winston with some details about her late husband. What do you think? Was that too little, just the right amount, or too much information? Did Dr. Konitz stumble on a tripping point?

When clients want to know about personal issues that may relate to the work you are doing, it can make sense to respond briefly and then remind clients of your professional training and experience. Some clients might persist and ask you to tell them more about yourself. There may be a couple of reasons for the persistence. One reason might be that they want a type of friendship in addition to the therapy relationship. Or they may be interested in your view on issues that concern them personally. A way to address the persistence is directly and honestly with a question like, "I appreciate your interest in my life and I am really interested in keeping our focus on your needs and thoughts."

Here are three examples of how therapists might address questions about a personal issue, such as being a parent: One therapist, coming from a psychoanalytic tradition (culture), might delay a direct answer and explore instead why the client is interested in how many children he has. He might say, "That's an interesting question. How would knowing about my children help our work together?" This comment or redirection is perfectly reasonable, because psychotherapy is all about exploring motives and the focus should stay on the client. For some therapists, this response may be too much of an assimilation strategy in that it doesn't allow what they would consider a respectful answering of the question. For others, it would be much more comfortable.

Another therapist might take a more existential or humanistic approach and respond, "I have two children. I'm wondering if my answer changes anything about our work together." Some therapists might consider this response more respectful. But notice that the focus is quickly brought back to the client.

Contrast these responses with a third psychotherapist, who may not be taking into account theoretical orientation or the focus of the session: "Oh! Let me show you pictures! Ronda is seven and Howard is two. Oh, they are so wonderful! Why, just yesterday …" In this interaction, the therapist might be choosing an extreme separation strategy or marginalization strategy.

Even though answering some questions from the client might be beneficial, the fragility of the therapeutic relationship makes self-disclosure a boundary issue. In psychotherapy, too much therapist self-disclosure introduces impurities into the relationship. Indeed, sometimes the less clients know about our private life, the better. Thus, we need to balance honesty and openness with other virtues, such as prudence and benevolence. For example, it is virtually never appropriate or useful for clients to hear about our current relationship struggles or financial hardships. One risk is that clients can interpret this type of sharing as an avenue to friendship. It can also switch the focus of a session, which can lead to compromising the primary reasons for therapy—client goals, growth, and wellbeing.

Your acculturation task is to find an appropriate response of honoring clients' desires to understand your personal experience while avoiding self-disclosure that compromises the work. As with all boundary issues, you need to consider variables such as the nature of the specific relationship, the client's gender, culture, age, and therapeutic goals, as well as your own values and tendencies.

Food for Thought: *Self-Disclosure*

How self-disclosive are you as a person? How detailed do you get when you tell stories? How much information do you share about yourself in your close relationships? In your more formal relationships?

It could be that you are very forthcoming and you sigh at the idea of not being able to be genuine with your clients. Even the notion that some disclosures may be less therapeutic than others is new to you! Or, it could be that you are more reserved—you've thought about therapy as a professional relationship that hinges on technique and not personality. Now you are encouraged to think about the possible benefits or ethical requirement that you disclose at least some information.

How do you think your "background level" of self-disclosure fits with the styles of the therapists described above? How might your preferences for self-disclosure fit within the different styles of psychotherapy that you know about?

For veteran therapists: How have your decisions about self-disclosure changed over the years? Why might that be?

Whether you are responding to clients' questions or sharing spontaneously, your self-disclosure runs the risk of diminishing the true focus of therapy. Thus, questions that move you toward integration are important to ask: Does your expertise and effectiveness come primarily from your personal life or from your professional training and experience? Does sharing information about your personal life lead to the best treatment outcomes (Foundation #1) and the most ethical behavior? How would you know it leads to the best treatment outcomes?

Another question to ask yourself when considering whether and how much to disclose is: Why would I share this information, with this client, at this time? Your desire to self-disclose is an indicator of some of your needs and motivations. For example, if you feel you want to disclose more about yourself to a particular client than to others, you can take that as a red flag about your needs and motivations, and perhaps a violation of beneficence and justice (Ethical Foundations #1 and #4) if your justification has more to do with your needs than the demands of the therapy. You might want to explore your possible attraction to the client. Your desire may be an indicator that your personal needs for connection are not being met elsewhere in your life.

Food for Thought: *Personal and Professional Considerations in Self-Disclosure*

Think back to Chapter 2 where you imagined your favorite and not so favorite client. Suppose you are in the session with your favorite client and they bring up a problem you recently or currently are facing in your life. On a scale from 1 to 10 (1 = not tempted at all; 10 = can't help myself), how tempted are you to disclose your own story? Here are some questions to consider:

- If I share my story (all or part), am I giving an example to show support or am I enjoying the experience of talking about myself?
- Can the focus of the session stay on the client or will it shift to me?
- Does the point of my story relate to the client's concerns?
- To what extent is the example helpful? To what extent would I just be rambling or bragging?

Now, rethink the situation: How might your thinking, feeling, and behavior change if the client is your least favorite client? See how your rating and the answers to the questions change. What might that mean?

Touching: A Physical and Psychological Boundary

Sexual touching between a therapist and client is never ethical. However, other types of touch warrant some careful deliberation. A pat on the back to one client might mean encouragement and support. However, another client might interpret it as a gesture of friendship, romance, or even as a sexual gesture. Depending on the culture, touch may be seen as a way to connect in the relationship. To "pull back physically, refuse a touch on the arm or a hug … might be alienating to the client" (Barnett, 2007, p. 403).

Some therapists take a very conservative view and avoid all touching. Other therapists will shake hands but do not go beyond that. These therapists see their approach as a way to show respect by treating clients equally (Foundation #4). After all, it is impossible to know how clients will react to behaviors like a hug or an arm around the shoulder. A client who has suffered sexual or physical abuse may see anything beyond a handshake as uncomfortable or harmful.

Clients' reactions to touch may also be related to their culture and family of origin. For example, some people grow up in families where physical touch is rare; it might be harder for them to avoid misinterpreting some forms of touch. Of course, therapists vary in their backgrounds as well. Some therapists may greet clients with a hug, or sometimes give a client a literal pat on the back. Therapists who choose this behavior may see it as a way to show warmth and caring as it was in their own families of origin, where everyone got hugs as they came and went.

Journal Entry: *To Touch or Not to Touch*

Of course, you can never know for sure how a particular client will receive your touch. However, you *can* assess your own intent. Write down 4–5 situations in which you might consider touching a client, in a variety of ways. Be specific about the situation, the characteristics of the client, and the type of touch. Then, consider these questions, for each scenario:

- Why would I touch this person at this time?
- What am I trying to communicate through my touch? What are some other ways to convey the same messages?
- What role does gender play in my decision about touching?
- To what extent am I influenced by whether the client is physically appealing to me?
- How do I touch?
- Have I asked the client if my touch is comfortable or uncomfortable?
- What situations, thoughts, emotions (i.e., tripping points) might lead me to make decisions that I know would be against my virtues or values?
- How might I evaluate whether my touch had the desired effect? How might my evaluation be biased?

Now, rethink each situation. How might your thinking, feeling, and behavior change if:

- The client was of a different gender or sexual orientation.
- The client's problem was about a religious issue.

- You were very attracted, physically, to the client.
- The client was of a different cultural group.
- You were being observed by a student therapist.
- You were being observed by a supervisor.

Journal Entry: *Tripping Points in Navigating Boundaries*

Sometimes we might be tempted to justify a behavior or protest too hard to make it feel more acceptable. Possibly a personal need is not being met, or our motivations are in conflict. It might also be that we are biased in our assessment of the situation—perhaps due to some acculturation stress.

Think about situations in your life where boundaries have changed or could change. Perhaps there have been times when you had difficulty in holding to boundaries. For example, you may lend money to friends, against your better judgment, to get them off your back or out of a sense of loyalty. Or you might have friends who don't respect your time—they are late to arrive or stay too long—and you haven't confronted them about it. Think about how these situations might be problematic with clients. For each situation, ask yourself questions like these to help determine whether such behaviors would be a boundary extension, crossing, or violation:

- What are your needs and motivations for changing the boundaries?
- Would there be an element of coercion or undue influence to change boundaries?
- Would there be any exploitation?
- With the change in boundaries, would roles still be maintained? If the boundary is changed back, would the roles revert back or are they changed for the long haul?
- How is culture and/or context influencing the change of boundaries?

Now, consider what tripping points might be hindering you in making your best choices:

- Although you believe your intentions to change boundaries are meant for good, how might your actions be perceived or inferred by others, such as members of the client's family, close colleagues of yours, and ethics committee members?

- What questions are you asking (and answering), and what more complex questions (and answers) might they be substituting for?
- How might you miss or misinterpret evidence for harm from your change of boundaries?

Inadvertent Contact

Boundary crossings happen accidentally: You see your client in a professional setting, in the grocery store or at a concert, your child is on the same soccer team as your client's child, or you happen to be guests at the same party. These situations happen, especially—but not only—in small communities. Is this a problem? It does not have to be, because you have choices about how to handle them.

Seeing a client at a concert, you would have the sense not to violate the therapeutic relationship by announcing, "Hey, look who's here—my favorite client!" On the other hand, clients may be really confused if you choose to ignore them all evening and act as if they are not even there. To prevent inadvertent contacts from being harmful (and even to provide some therapeutic benefit), it is important for you and your clients to discuss the situation in therapy.

When you anticipate that inadvertent contact is likely to occur (for example, in small communities), you can talk about it with your client beforehand and decide how you want to handle the situation. One good approach is the *You First* arrangement (Knapp et al., 2017). Using the You First strategy, you will leave it up to the client to initiate contact, say hello, introduce you to others, or whatever. If the client does not initiate, then no contact or no recognition occurs. This is a good arrangement because clients maintain control over the situation; you have respected their autonomy. In fact, this could be one the points discussed during the informed consent process (see Chapter 7).

Time Boundaries

In our opening story, Mr. Desmond recognized Greta's pattern of becoming more emotional as the end of the session came closer. Mr. Desmond would let the session go on longer and eventually would stand up to begin to usher Greta out of the room so that he could meet with his next client. Time can be a difficult boundary to navigate. Clients may genuinely need a little extra time, and we don't like the feeling of shutting people down emotionally. This can be especially true for new therapists. Think back to your list of motivations for entering the field. Do any of your motivations, or your needs and values, suggest that holding this boundary might be difficult? Also think about your most and least favorite clients: Might you treat these two people differently when it comes to time? Depending on your responses to these questions, you might need to strengthen your boundaries in this area.

Gifts

Decisions regarding gifts from clients include deliberation of several variables, including context, culture, the value of the gift, the nature of the therapy, the time in the therapeutic relationship, client and therapist motivations and expectations, and the potential meaning of the gift (Lazarus, 2007; Vasquez, 2007). Vasquez provides an example of a client who brings her therapist a taco to eat because the session was at noon and the therapist squeezed her in due to a crisis. Vasquez concludes that "sometimes a taco is just a taco" (2007, p. 407) and the therapist should recognize the gift as a culturally accepted way of expressing gratitude—a boundary extension.

On the other hand, an expensive gift, or a pattern of gift giving from a client, could become a boundary violation, and needs to be explored with the client. This exploration of the client's expectations or motivations might lead to some important benefits for the client. Could it be that the client feels they need to bring some type of gift to equalize the relationship, or see the gift as a way to increase their value in the relationship? These are worthy issues to explore.

Social Media

In Chapter 3, we introduced the issue of patient-targeted googling (Reinert & Kowacs, 2019). The internet is a relatively new way to get information about our clients (and for our clients to get information about us!). One of the major questions is this: How do we respect our clients' right to autonomy? In the session, clients share what they want us to know, nothing more and nothing less at that time. On social media or the internet, we might access information they have chosen not to share with us. We might also find information that contradicts what they have shared in session. This kind of knowledge can impede our ability to work with our clients.

Perspectives on Multiple Relationships

Multiple relationships are ongoing boundary crossings or violations that develop into identifiable relationships. Here is a short list of possible multiple relationships:

- Being a therapist for a friend, relative, employee, and/or student.
- Developing a friendship with a client.
- Being members within the same professional organization.
- Becoming an evaluator, such as doing a custody evaluation for a client's child.
- Entering into a business venture (other than the therapy, of course) with a client.
- Entering into therapy with a person with whom you have had sexual relations.

Similar to self-disclosure and other boundary issues, there is a lively debate and a continuum of perspectives about the ethical nature of multiple relationships with clients. Although there is general agreement about sexual relationships with current clients, some authors see other multiple relationships (e.g., friendships with clients or being a dental patient of your client) as appropriate, ethical, and just the way life is or should be (Lazarus, 2007; Lazarus & Zur, 2002; Speight, 2012). The question to be addressed is "which multiple relationships are never appropriate, which ones are acceptable, and which ones must be engaged in" (Barnett, 2007, p. 403).

Kitchener (2000) has written a lot about multiple relationships and their problematic nature, and takes a conservative approach. This is the way she explains it: In every relationship, people play roles, and each role has a set of expectations (what others think we should do or be like) and a set of obligations (those things required of us). Consistent with our role expectations and obligations, we act in ways that ensure clients' wellbeing (Foundation #1), that respect their confidences (Foundation #7), and we maintain boundaries (Foundation #6). Entering into another type of relationship introduces a whole new set of role expectations and obligations. These new expectations and obligations can compromise the therapeutic ones. Therapists can experience role strain and clients can experience disequilibrium.

Consider the case of friendship: Both parties and their personal needs are of equal importance in a friendship. Both parties engage in similar amounts of self-disclosure, and both parties feel free to give and receive advice. In therapy, the relationship is much more asymmetrical. Clients who are also friends may very likely feel frustrated, confused, and angry trying to make sense of the role changes.

When a therapy relationship turns into another one, it can be difficult or impossible to turn back the clock and go back to *just* the therapy role. The dynamics (expectations, obligations, power) of the other relationship are still present and potentially harmful to the therapy relationship. Multiple relationships can stem from simple boundary crossings and other behaviors, which are well represented among our red flags! They do not seem dramatic at the time, but they still compromise the purity and integrity of the therapy relationship.

Even When Therapy Is Over, the Relationship Lives on

At this point you might be thinking, "OK, I see your point about multiple relationships during therapy. But what about when therapy is over? We can be friends (or lovers, or business partners, or …), right?"

Relationships don't stop on a dime. Research (Anderson & Kitchener, 1996; Buckley et al., 1981) suggests that aspects of the therapeutic relationship continue for clients. Thus, sequential multiple relationships can be as problematic as simultaneous ones. If you have done some good work with clients, they may want to resume therapy in the future. (As we mentioned before, switching back to a therapy relationship is hard, or impossible.)

The temptation to initiate another relationship with your client or former client can be a serious tripping point. This might be a perfect time to invoke the *Why Bother Rule*. That is: Why bother doing something ethically questionable or problematic when you might be opening the door to potential harms? Anderson and Kitchener (1998) state it this way: "The greater the risk of an adverse consequence, such as undermining the trust established or the gains made in a psychotherapy relationship, the greater the need to avoid entering into the relationship" (p. 93). Good therapy is a great accomplishment and a big investment on both sides. Why complicate things and disrupt what you have accomplished?

Unavoidable Multiple Relationships

Of course, there are times when multiple relationships with clients are unavoidable. For example, you and your client (or former client) might find yourselves on the same committee at your child's school or part of the same social/professional network. When this happens, clarity about how to handle this other relationship for the benefit of the client is of utmost importance. As a minimum, you and your client need to talk through how to manage this additional relationship. How will the two of you handle confidentiality? How will you work to keep the roles compartmentalized to minimize possible harm? What steps will you or your client take if roles do get confusing and either or both of you are concerned about the new roles? Bottom line: It is important to make good acculturation choices, recognizing your professional obligations, personal values and motivations, and the likelihood of harm (Anderson & Kitchener, 1998).

Green Flag: *Responsible Referrals*

Here is an example of a psychotherapist practicing good reflection about the possibility of taking on another role with a client. After you read this scenario, speculate about the acculturation influences and choices of Dr. Ruiz:

> Norah is seeing Dr. Ruiz and the therapy is going well. Dr. Ruiz notices that Norah is talking about different kinds of life choices, career issues, time management, and stuff that could really be done by coaching rather than therapy. Dr. Ruiz considers switching from therapy to coaching, and offering Norah her coaching skills. After all, she's been trained to be a coach in addition to her therapy training. But then Dr. Ruiz has two thoughts that save her and Norah from a boundary violation. First, Dr. Ruiz thinks, "Wait; if I do coaching, it'll get in the way of our good therapy work." Second, Dr.

Ruiz thinks, "Why am I so arrogant as to think that I am the only person who can provide coaching to Norah?" Using an ethics frame in addition to a therapy or coaching frame, Dr. Ruiz concludes that switching relationships might feel coercive to Norah and consequently infringe upon her autonomy. The switch might not work out, and thus violate the principles of beneficence and nonmaleficence.

At the end of the next session, Dr. Ruiz says, "Norah, I notice that there are some issues you are talking about that might be well suited to explore with a life coach. Here is a list of three local people who do life coaching. You may want to think about that option."

Norah says, "But, Dr. Ruiz, you are trained as a life coach, right?"

"Yes."

"So, why can't you coach me? You already know a lot about me," Norah asks, reasonably.

Just a faint touch of a smile crosses Dr. Ruiz's face as she thinks to herself, "In graduate school they said I'd get questions like this from clients, and I didn't believe them!" Out loud, she says, "Norah, although there are similarities between psychotherapy and coaching, they are still different and if we switched to do that, I can't guarantee that the therapy we've been working so hard at would be as good. It's a much better idea, I think, if we keep working like we have been, and you see somebody who can devote all their energies to coaching. Does that make sense? Think about working with a life coach; there's no need to make up your mind right now."

Conclusion

Boundaries are a real and very complex issue in all therapy relationships. Boundary violations are never ethical. There are times when we need to say clearly to our clients: "No thank you. I just want to be your therapist." However, sometimes we decide to extend or cross boundaries to do our best for clients. For example, issues of culture and context may make an extension or crossing desirable. But we always make such decisions mindfully, not intuitively. Examination of needs, motivations, and values is imperative, as is understanding and accounting for red flags and tripping points. Once again, we are more likely to achieve ethical excellence when we are drawing upon our core and our professional guides, and we are moving toward integration strategies.

6

Confidentiality
A Critical Element of Trust in the Relationship

Clients take risks in therapy by sharing intimate details of their lives. To take those risks, clients need to trust therapists to keep those details private. With this being the case, we might say that confidentiality—the promise of privacy—is a foundation of our mansion. It is the cornerstone of the therapy relationship—all other stones occupy their positions in reference to this stone. Without that explicit and implicit promise—"I will keep your information confidential"—the trustworthiness of the therapist is not a viable possibility. Thus, keeping the confidences of clients is one of the major role obligations of psychotherapists and a hallmark of the culture of psychotherapy. As you might suspect, however, the concept is not absolute and not as simple as it first appears.

Confidentiality is both an ethical and legal concept. All the professional codes address the issue of confidentiality and many states have laws that identify the term *legal confidentiality*, which mandates that conversations between a client and psychotherapist cannot be shared with another individual without legal ramifications (Cottone & Tarvydas, 2016).

Sensitivity and Understanding of Confidentiality

Personal—Your Core and Pre-existing Culture About Confidentiality

Before we go any further, let's look at your core and at aspects of your pre-existing "confidentiality culture" with an eye toward deciding which aspects will be worth maintaining and which may be incompatible with the culture of psychotherapy.

Journal Entry: *Me and Secrets*

We encourage you to think and write about four actual or potential situations from your life.

First Situation: Consider a time when you told someone something very personal, expecting them to keep the information to themselves. However, they didn't keep your secret—they told another person or they put it on social media. If you cannot think of a particular instance, speculate about an incident that could have happened in your life. Answer these questions:

- Who was (or would be) that person you shared your secret with and what is their relationship with you?
- How does (would) it feel to have your personal information shared by this person?
- What (might have) happened to your relationship with them?

Second Situation: Consider a time when you shared personal information with someone else and (at least to the best of your knowledge) they kept your secret.

- Who was (is) the person you trusted with the secret?
- What prompted you to trust them?
- What was (is) the relationship like with that person?
- What was (is) it about that person, do you think, that helps them honor your confidences?
- Write about some of the similarities and differences between your first two situations. You might write about the context, the relationships, your feelings, or the other persons' motives for sharing or keeping your secret.

Third Situation: Let's turn the tables and have you reflect about yourself in the "secret keeper" role. Write about a time when someone shared something personal with you and they expected you to keep their confidence but you ended up sharing the information with a third party.

- Who were the people, and what was (is) their relationship with you?
- What happened or what prompted you to share the information?
- What did it feel like to make and carry out the decision? (If you feel like you shared the information without a conscious decision, we encourage you to think again!)

- What happened to the relationship between you and the person whose confidence you shared?
- Why were you not able to keep this secret?

Fourth Situation: Write about a time when you kept a secret that was told to you by somebody, even when you experienced some temptation to share it. Write the story and then answer these questions:

- To whom were you tempted to tell the information?
- Why were you tempted?
- What did it feel like to keep the confidence?
- What did you draw upon from your core that enabled you to keep the secret this time around?
- What is the relationship like now?

We make decisions every day about what personal information of ours we want to share with others and the kinds of information that others have shared with us. Many of the decisions we make are second nature; we may not even realize that we have rules about what to share with whom, when. Your answers in this journal entry provide some important information about the personal rules you have—what's in your core—regarding maintaining privacy or keeping secrets. Knowing these rules makes you better prepared to protect your clients' confidentiality in therapy.

Here's another exercise: Identify a specific person in each of the categories of people below. If you can't—you don't have an attorney, for example—think about another person who plays a similar role in your life (e.g., your accountant).

- A parent
- A distant cousin
- An acquaintance
- Your closest friend
- Your spouse/partner/significant other
- Your attorney
- Your physician
- Your clergyperson

Now, think about some types of personal information you would or would not share with each of these people. For example, to whom among the above individuals and under what conditions might you tell them:

- your hopes and dreams for the future;
- a store you shop at that you are a little embarrassed about;

- an incident in childhood that you'd rather forget;
- a sexual behavior or position you've always wanted to try but haven't.

Now, consider each of these people telling you these things. How might you react?

Your sensitivity to issues of privacy and confidentiality is an important place to start, for several reasons. First, dilemmas and issues revolving around confidentiality are among the most common dilemmas therapists face (Pettifor, 2004; Pope & Vetter, 1992).

Second, many of our students—and some professionals already in the field—give us the impression that their core ideas about privacy are usually *not* enough to honor fully the principle of confidentiality in psychotherapy. For example, during a class discussion on confidentiality, Sharon remembers a student being very honest and saying, "This keeping secrets and confidentiality thing will really be tough. I am naturally nosy and I like to share good stories." We suspect that laid-back attitudes about confidentiality may be more common in today's world of the internet and social media. A picture, comment, or opinion can more easily become visible to whoever has the interest and diligence to search the internet. Sometimes, just the slip of a finger on the "send" button or not verifying the correct recipient results in violating client confidentiality. Even in this world of immediate access to personal information, however, psychotherapists have the obligation to uphold the promise of confidentiality to provide that safe space for clients.

The third reason to develop and maintain our sensitivity is that people in our personal lives may be used to us sharing our experiences of the day; they (and we!) may value this as a way to stay close and connected. Valuing our new professional obligations and negotiating shifts in our personal relationships is a major acculturation task.

Fourth, culture and context influence the parameters and understanding of confidentiality. For collective cultures, the circle of confidentiality and the work in therapy may include family members or others who need or have a right to know.

Finally, there are times when confidentiality must be breached. The promise of confidentiality in therapy is not and cannot be absolute. There are times when, for the client's or someone else's safety, therapists must share confidential information. No matter how experienced they are, breaking the client's confidentiality, when it is ethically and legally necessary, can be one of the more heart-wrenching and uncomfortable tasks psychotherapists face.

Professional—Confidentiality in the Psychotherapy Culture

To provide the opportunity to have clients say anything at all—no matter how embarrassing or deeply personal—and have the statements valued, respected, and protected from disclosure is a "sacred covenant" (Driscoll, 1992, p. 704) between us and our clients. Our obligation is based in part on the constitutional right of privacy—you and I have the right to decide who knows what about us when (Kitchener & Anderson, 2011). In addition, the critical role of confidentiality for therapy to be effective was highlighted in a ground-breaking case by the Supreme Court of the United States, Jaffee v. Redmond (1996). As Younggren and Harris (2008) state, our duty "to protect the client's privacy comes from the fiduciary nature of the professional relationship" (p. 590).

In today's world of immediate access to information, the privacy of psychotherapy may be even more special. Thus, the obligation to uphold our promise and provide that safe space for clients may be more important than ever. However, clients may feel a push-pull and some confusion about our promise of confidentiality. On one hand, they want to accept the offer of confidentiality fully—to trust the therapist—and be able to share themselves without any hesitation. On the other hand, they may be unfamiliar with such promises and fear the possibility that the therapist will (a) judge the personal information that they hear; (b) disclose the clients' confidences to colleagues, spouses, or others; or (c) somehow allude to their personal information on the internet. They may have a history with close relationships where their confidences were disrespected.

Welfel (2016) makes the important point that *everything* said between a client and a therapist is confidential, no matter how dull or routine it might be, and no matter how good it might be as a story for your next get-together with friends or family. What we might consider mundane, ordinary, and unnecessary to keep as a confidence, clients might see as very private, personal parts of themselves. Welfel (2016) connects confidentiality to virtue (Foundation #8):

> Zealously guarding client privacy also indicates a true compassion for the courage it takes for clients to enter treatment … Honoring confidentiality requires integrity precisely because it can be difficult—the human tendency to want to share experiences does not bypass mental health professionals simply because they have a credential. (p. 114)

We have heard something like this from more than one student: "Wow, I tell my partner everything. It's a very important part of our relationship. You mean, now I have to keep secrets from them?" Our response is, "Yes, absolutely!" You need to set and keep a boundary with significant others in your life about client confidentiality. Your spouse, partner, and best friends are not supposed to be the benefactors of interesting stories from clients. Nor are they entitled to be privy to that level or type of detail about your work.

Psychotherapists whose core might be less sensitized and who choose a separation strategy might argue, "Come on. My client tells me about their favorite department store and this is supposed to be confidential? It won't do any harm to share that information with my spouse!" Although it seems picky and extreme not to be able to share such a trivial tidbit, a promise of confidentiality is a promise of confidentiality. It is true that the risk of harm is quite low in this example, but the underlying principle goes beyond doing good (Foundation #1) and avoiding harm (Foundation #2) to Foundation #3: "Respect clients' autonomy." Bok (1989) encourages us to remember that keeping our promise with the small and trivial issues shows the client that we can be trusted with the more important matters they disclose. She also says that maintaining confidentiality expresses our virtues (Foundation #8), including diligence, prudence, and integrity.

Although there are exceptions to confidentiality, which we discuss shortly, the default option is keeping everything a client says confidential unless there is a clear reason to disclose the information, rather than picking and choosing what we perceive as interesting stories from our clients as possible material for our next dinner conversation. Clients often assume that what they share is confidential. They don't feel the need to stop and say, "You'll keep this just between the two of us, right?" which is what typically happens between friends or colleagues at work. Thus, you may want to think of your obligation this way: There are no trivial disclosures.

Confidentiality in therapy extends all the way to revealing a client's identity (Welfel, 2016), which is called *contact confidentiality* (Ahia & Martin, 1993). As psychotherapists we have the obligation to keep our clients' identities unknown to others. The following story is an example of (among other problems) not honoring a client's identity.

Red Flags: *Compromised Confidentiality and Overlooked Oppression*

> Dr. Bechet is dedicated to helping people. One day he says to one of his clients, Mr. Armstrong, "I know we have been talking about how you want to meet people and how it's difficult being … your race and all. I was wondering. Have you thought about the internet—like online dating? One of my other clients, Pat, is trying it out. It seems to be a good avenue. The two of you might even come across each other's profile. You have some things in common."
>
> "I don't—" says Mr. Armstrong, deciding whether he is more upset about the race comment or the assumption of a therapist suggesting online dating to meet people.
>
> "Oh, give it a try. I'll text the url to you. Oh, and Pat's last name is Smith."
> Mr. Armstrong hears the alert on his phone—text received.

Dr. Bechet is definitely not maintaining confidentiality and his lack of cultural sensitivity seems apparent. We might not be as culturally insensitive or cross the confidentiality boundary as blatantly as Dr. Bechet, but even the small things like talking to clients in the hallway or waiting area indicates that we may not be actualizing the true essence or promise of confidentiality.

Food for Thought: *The Red Flag of Porous Privacy*

We use the term *porous privacy* for when therapists compromise confidentiality by sharing information about one client with another individual or individuals without consent. Like other violations of confidentiality, porous privacy is disrespectful (Foundation #3) and potentially harmful (Foundation #2). Porous privacy sometimes takes the form of bragging—for example, the therapist who loves to tell stories about her therapeutic triumphs, or our therapist in Chapter 1 who was tempted to tell others that they were the "shrink" referred to by a successful comedian. The most problematic version of this behavior is a full disclosure, with names and/or other identifying information about some experience of clients. Thus, it is very important to be open about your motivations as you look at your own judgments and behaviors regarding privacy. This might sound flippant, but we say it this way for emphasis: If you want something to brag about, you might want to join a bowling league or sew quilts in your spare time.

The following are some vignettes for exploration:

Chris didn't think much about the first of the following comments by his therapist, Dr. Pizzarelli. But by the third one, the pattern was clear, and Chris felt he should have seen the threat to his own privacy coming.

1. Dr. Pizzarelli leaned in a little toward Chris and said, "I just used this approach with another client of mine. Her partner was just written up in the paper for that big accident—it was all over the news. It was horrible."
2. Patting Chris on the arm, Dr. Pizzarelli sounded sympathetic, "It's not unusual to feel that way. Steve, who was my last appointment, went through the same thing a month ago. Thought he might have to quit his job at the community college."
3. Handing Chris a card, Dr. Pizzarelli announced, "You mentioned last week that you were thinking about changing your life insurance. I have a friend

who's a broker. When I told him about you, he said he'd be happy to help. He'll be calling you by the end of the week."

Part 1.   Put yourself in the position of Chris.

- What are your reactions as you listen to Dr. Pizzarelli make the first two comments?
- How would you feel when it occurred to you that Dr. Pizzarelli might be talking about you to other clients?

Part 2.   You are the member of the State Regulatory Board for psychotherapists. Chris files a complaint with the Board. He charges that Dr. Pizzarelli has violated the confidentiality of himself and other clients. Other clients have also filed complaints about Dr. Pizzarelli's breaches of confidentiality. The State Board is charged with investigating these complaints, deciding if a violation of confidentiality has occurred, and if so, deciding on a suitable punishment or remedial plan depending on the seriousness of the violation. As a Board member:

- Do you feel that confidentiality has been violated?
- On a scale from 1 to 10, with 1 being helpful and 10 being horrendous, where would you rate Dr. Pizzarelli's behavior? Why?
- Was any harm done? (Refer back to the questions in Part 1.)
- What kind of discipline or punishment, if any, should Dr. Pizzarelli receive?

Part 3.   Put yourself in the position of Dr. Pizzarelli:

- Why did you say the things you did? Think of both appropriate and inappropriate motivations. Think about the personal values you might be drawing upon. Think of the tripping points that you may have missed.
- How could you have gotten the same therapeutic impact without providing information about other clients?
- What if you said the same things about a client (or conveyed the same information about a client) to a close friend over lunch, a colleague with whom you were consulting, or a partner as you went to bed and were sharing your day with each other?

Part 4.   Finally, play with this scenario a little bit. Change the context of the service (rural or small community), genders, ethnic backgrounds, ages, and other characteristics of the client, the psychotherapist, and the Board members. How do these changes influence your thinking?

Can We Ever Say ANYTHING?

Is there anything we can say to others about what we do in psychotherapy without violating our promise? As we discussed in Chapter 3, people will ask you things like, "How'd it go today?" We cannot violate our promise of confidentiality, but neither are we expected to totally sacrifice our own personalities, mental health, and relationships. We need to draw upon our core and work out some assimilation and integration strategies.

One common way to handle this situation is to talk about our experiences and feelings as a therapist without sharing identities or personal information of our clients. For example, we can talk to our significant others about how splendidly our day went and share the joys and frustrations of being a therapist—without the detail on which these reactions are based. We can talk to colleagues about various types of clients who don't connect well with, or who frustrate, us. However, if we need consultation on a particular case, to talk about issues such as different worldviews or cultural identities, or diagnostic issues, we would need either to get the permission of our clients to get that consultation or to refrain from revealing identifying information (APA, 2017, Standard 4.06).

Sometimes both the therapist and client agree that information from therapy should be shared with others, including physicians and other professionals, work supervisors, clients' family members, and others. The client has the power to give us permission to talk with others (APA, 2017, Standard 4.05). In these cases, we get our clients' written permission to share information with appropriate professionals. That is, they waive their right to confidentiality through signing a *Release of Information* form that specifies who is involved, what kinds of information we can share, and for how long we have that permission.

Green Flags: *Effective Ethical Explanations and Requests for Written Releases*

As you read this story, think about the virtues Dr. Tall is displaying:

"Have you been in mental health treatment before?" Dr. Tall asks Jane.

"Oh, yes; I saw a psychiatrist last year for medication. But I didn't like the side effects."

"I think it would be a good idea if I talked to your former psychiatrist. I would also like to talk with your physician, given the physical complaints you have."

"Sure! Talk with any of those folks. I'll give you their names and numbers."

"That's great; I'll just need you to sign a couple of release forms. It'll only take a few minutes."

Jane fidgets a bit in her chair. "Oh, we don't need forms. I already gave you my permission, and I trust you."

Dr. Tall is not fazed. "It's more than a matter of trust. The forms help to refresh our memories and also give you the opportunity to change your mind."

"So, what exactly am I signing?"

"This form says that I can share information with your psychiatrist for purposes of your treatment. That means I won't just gossip! And the expiration date is six months from today, so if I need to talk with her after that, I'll ask you to renew your permission."

"And you said I could change my mind?"

"Sure. For any reason. It usually doesn't happen, but you have that right. Just tell me you don't want me to talk to her any more, and I'll make a note in your chart. And, by the way, we'll fill one of these out for each person, and I'll give you a copy of each of the forms, so you know what permissions you gave."

There are other situations in which sharing some information may be acceptable. For example, when we teach we often use examples of cases we see for instructional purposes. The professions recognize the importance of teaching and the importance of using examples that capture the reality of therapy (APA, 2017, Standard 4.07). We are allowed, therefore, to use our clinical case material as illustrations. However, we must carefully and fully disguise the identities of our clients (or, of course, get their permission, which is often clinically contraindicated).

Food for Thought: *To Breach or Not to Breach*

Once upon a time there was a psychotherapist, Dr. D. Lemmah, who had been seeing a female client, Elaine, for several months. Elaine was gaining some wonderful insights into her history of failed relationships. One day Elaine comes into the session with a little smile on her face. She sits down and immediately tells Dr. Lemmah about this new person in her life, Jerry. They've been on a couple dates and things are going quite well. She really thinks she's made some improvement in being more open and vulnerable! As she shares more detail about Jerry, Dr. Lemmah notices a slight ringing in the ears along with an uneasy feeling that starts in the head and travels down to the abdomen, and finally settles as a definite sinking feeling in the stomach. Jerry was a client of Dr. Lemmah's, having terminated two years ago. Jerry had made some progress with depression and anxiety, but Dr. Lemmah remembers that Jerry had been charged with a felony—physically abusing an ex-partner.

Consider the following questions. Be as explicit as you can in your responses:

- What are your thoughts about and feelings toward Dr. Lemmah, Elaine, and Jerry? With whom do you identify the most? What gender did you assume for Dr. Lemmah? What gender did you assume for Jerry?
- If you were not Elaine's therapist and you had the same information about Jerry, what would you tell Elaine? Why?

Put yourself in Dr. Lemmah's place:

1. What are your ethical obligations to Elaine? To Jerry? To your profession?
2. What are your options for how to proceed?
3. How tempted are you to breach Jerry's confidentiality? Not at all, kind of, absolutely? Why? What frame(s) are you using? What other tripping points might be present?
4. What do you decide to do? Why?
5. What facts of the case would have to be different for you to choose other options?

Put yourself in Jerry's place:

6. What would you expect Dr. Lemmah to do in this case? Why?

Put yourself in Elaine's place:

7. What would you expect Dr. Lemmah to do in this case? Why?
8. How might you feel about Dr. Lemmah's decision?

Put yourself in the place of an ethics committee member:

9. The committee receives a complaint about Dr. Lemmah from Elaine, who recently broke up with Jerry and Elaine was physically harmed. During their breakup, it became apparent that Jerry was a former client of Dr. Lemmah, and Elaine was furious that Dr. Lemmah did not tell her about Jerry weeks before. She believes Dr. Lemmah acted unethically by not informing her of his knowledge about Jerry and insisting that she break up with Jerry immediately. What does the committee decide and on what grounds?
10. The committee receives a complaint about Dr. Lemmah from Jerry, with whom Elaine recently broke up. During their breakup, it became apparent that Elaine was a client of Dr. Lemmah and that he strongly suggested that

Elaine end her relationship with Jerry. Jerry is furious. Jerry believes Dr. Lemmah acted unethically by breaching client confidentiality and incompetently by telling Elaine what to do rather than simply exploring her decisions. What does the committee decide and on what grounds?

Work through all these questions (1–10) again under the following conditions:

- Jerry is a person of color. If truth be known, you harbor some uncomfortable feelings toward Jerry's racial group.
- Elaine is now Edward. What gender did you assume for Jerry? Depending on your answer, how does the gender of each of them affect your gut reactions and professional judgments?
- Elaine is a transgender woman and Jerry is a cisgender man. How does the identity of transgender affect your gut reactions and professional judgments?

Final Questions:

- What conflicts (of motives, values, virtues, and principles) were the most salient for you?
- What did you notice from your core and from integrating your ethics of origin and your professional responsibilities? For example, did you reorganize your values to allow one to become more prominent? Did you shift your ideas about how to implement your values?

Limits to Confidentiality

There are times when therapists cannot and should not maintain confidentiality. The promise to respect clients' confidences comes with exceptions that need to be conveyed to clients in clear terms at the start of the therapy relationship. (We'll cover more about this in Chapter 7.) These exceptions revolve around the safety of clients and/or others.

Respecting client autonomy (Foundation #3; Kitchener & Anderson, 2011) means (among other things) that clients have the right to choose who will know what about them when. However, the right to such autonomy is limited when that right infringes the rights of others. For example, if a client indicates in therapy that a child is being abused (and, in some states, an elder is being abused), state laws require the therapist to report such abuse. If a client is planning to kill another individual, the psychotherapist has the ethical—and in most states, the legal—responsibility to warn the potential victim of the possible harm and to take other steps to protect the potential victim, such as contacting the police and getting the client hospitalized for a psychiatric evaluation (*Tarasoff*, 1976). Likewise, if a client threatens to kill himself or herself, therapists are obligated to break confidentiality to save the client's life.

Breaching confidentiality to report abuse of a minor or elder, prevent a murder, or stop a suicide are clear instances of overriding a client's privacy for the purpose of preventing a terrible harm. But let's take this opportunity to explore potentially difficult situations where you think confidentiality might need to be breached.

Journal Entry: *Once More into the Breach*

For each of the following situations, answer these questions: (a) What is your gut feeling about what you would *like* to do in each case? (b) Does your course of action involve a breach of confidentiality? (c) What courses of action are possible? (d) What does the profession (according to your other texts, professor, colleagues, ethics code) think about whether you should violate confidentiality? (e) What would you choose to do and why (consider your core, virtues, values, and so forth? (f) What tripping points might make it hard for you to make and carry through with a good decision?

In therapy, a client tells you that they:

1. are feeling sad and sometimes wish for death;
2. are really angry with a former partner;
3. are having an affair;
4. have robbed a store;
5. plan to embezzle money from the bank that employs them;
6. plan to embezzle money from the bank that employs them and which happens to be *your* bank;
7. drink or do drugs and are underage;
8. engaged in touching children sexually;
9. have engaged in touching children sexually 30 years ago, but don't any more;
10. have tested positive for HIV and are having unprotected sex.

Now look at your answers. Which situations prompted the most discomfort? What virtues, principles, ethics codes, and other sources of guidance did you call upon to make your professional decisions? What dimensions and tripping points stand out, as you look at the pattern of your responses, in your decision making? Was it only that some harm was done? The type of harm (e.g., physical vs. financial)? The amount of harm? The imminence of the harm? What happened when children were involved?

The limits on, or exceptions to, confidentiality are prescribed by state statute, case law, and administrative law. In most states, homicidal threats are grounds for violating confidentiality, as are threats of suicide. All states have laws about reporting child abuse, although they vary regarding the specific professionals required to report and some of the parameters of such reporting. For example, in some states the situation in #9 in the previous journal entry would have to be reported—in other states, not. Some states require reporting of elder abuse, others do not. States also vary about whether minors are guaranteed confidentiality.

In addition to laws, agencies have their own policies about confidentiality. In an important sense, each agency represents a mini-culture, with its own codes, traditions, and values.

Food for Thought: *Spouse/Partner Abuse*

Do you think spouse or partner abuse ought to be a reportable offense? That is, if you find out that one person in the relationship is physically abusive, should you report that to the authorities? Justify your answer in terms of ethics through motivations, values, virtues, principles, and so forth. Then, justify an *opposing* point of view.

The acculturation tasks regarding the limits of confidentiality may be quite stressful. How are we to move toward integration? Some of you may feel that these exceptions are too much—therapy should be treated as sacred; psychotherapists cannot take on police functions (Siegel, 1979). Indeed, coming to therapy where you are guaranteed a place to work out your problems in total privacy may actually reduce the total number of crimes committed in the population (this argument was in the minority opinion in the *Tarasoff* [1976] decision). Those of you with these types of beliefs might adopt a separation strategy and be rather slow to breach confidentiality even when such an action is obligatory, as in the case of child abuse.

Another possible response to learning of these exceptions to confidentiality is that the exceptions do not go far enough! You might be among those whose ordinary moral sense would suggest reporting a robbery or embezzlement by your clients. However, robbery and embezzlement do *not* need to be reported; therefore, breaking confidentiality to report them would be unethical.

It may be difficult to violate confidentiality even when it is clearly justified. Indeed, many therapists report difficulty—acculturation stress, if you will—when dealing with these issues (Pope & Vetter, 1992). When the situation or conversation suggests that we must violate confidentiality—even when we've told our clients the limits of our promise—our minds and hearts feel the conflict acutely. Our need to reduce the ambiguity inherent in such situations may prompt us to make precipitous—and wrong—decisions. As we consider how violating confidentiality might affect the relationship, other tripping points might ensue, such as ethical fading.

How do we choose integration strategies that encourage us to preserve confidentiality in most situations and violate confidentiality appropriately in others? One general strategy is to keep four thoughts in mind. First, the way we implement our ethical obligation, whether it is to violate or preserve confidentiality, is critical. Second, the welfare of the client (or the intended victim of a serious threat, or the child in the case of child abuse) may be the highest principle. Third, we may not be the final arbiters—or providers—of that welfare. Fourth, consultation is an important action to pursue. Consultation, peer supervision, and other ways to share and get feedback on your professional decisions can really help. Indeed, in many states the failure to get consultation itself constitutes unprofessional conduct.

It's a Small World After All

Sometimes confidentiality is compromised through no fault of our own. Our world is smaller than we think; there may be times when we accidently end up seeing our client in a grocery store, in a gym, or at a concert. Our child may wind up on the same athletic team as our client's child, or we happen to be guests at the same party. Sometimes we are part of a small community, geographically or culturally. How we handle our client's confidentiality in these situations is important and communicates to the client our respect for the professional relationship. It is important to discuss these possible events occurring and decide how to handle them, such as the "You First" arrangement (Knapp et al., 2017; see Chapter 5).

Privilege and Confidentiality

Sometimes psychotherapists use the terms *privilege* and *confidentiality* interchangeably in casual conversation (Welfel, 2016). In actuality, they are two different terms and come from two very different cultures. *Privilege* and *privileged communication* are exclusively legal terms. Privilege is the right of the (adult) client to keep any communication that occurs in therapy from being revealed *in legal proceedings* (Cottone & Tarvydas, 2016).

Similar to confidentiality, the right of privileged communication has limitations. In a civil proceeding, the judge can issue a court order to have a therapist share information or produce client records. At this point, of course, prudent therapists get legal consultation to help them navigate this new culture. Psychotherapists and their attorneys can file appeals to the ruling, they can request that a higher court hear the psychotherapist's assertion of privileged communication, or the psychotherapist can decide to deal with the legal ramifications of refusing to cooperate with the court order.

We leave you with one more scenario.

Red Flags: *Logistical Laxity and Porous Privacy*

Consider this from a friend or acquaintance: My daughter and I are seeing a child/ family psychologist. It's like our fourth or fifth visit, and he's in a practice with other people, so they have this common waiting room. My daughter and I get there and we're sittin' in the lobby area. And there's three other people waiting for their therapist. He comes out, you know, and says, "Is there anything I need to know about your daughter?"'cause he's gonna work with my daughter. This doesn't feel so good. So I just kind of give him some general stuff, you know, in front of these three other people I don't know!

My daughter leaves with him and all of a sudden it hits me. Wow, that guy's violating my daughter's privacy. Why couldn't we have taken a couple of minutes to talk in his office? I laughed a little, like, I should know these things—I'm a mental health professional myself! Why didn't I say something? But it's different. Now I'm on the client side.

When I got home, I called the therapist and left a voice message and said, "It didn't feel real good when you asked the question, 'Is there anything I need to know about your daughter?' out in the lobby. I want to be able to go back in your office and address whatever I need to. That's the usual process."

He called back the next day and said, "Well, I hope you didn't see that as unprofessional behavior." In my head, I'm thinking, "Yeah! I did! Because it was!"

He said, "I didn't mean for you to disclose anything you wouldn't want to." I responded with, "From now on I would prefer we discuss my daughter's progress in your office and not in front of others. It's a little extra effort but that's important."

As you read this story, what thoughts and feelings come up in you for the daughter who's the client? For the narrator of the story? For the psychologist who is seeing the client?

7

Informed Consent
The Three-Legged Stool

"Knowledge is power."
Sir Francis Bacon

Our opening story comes from Mitch:

> When I was a kid, my older brother used to ask me all the time if I wanted to play Monopoly. I always said, "Sure!" I was just learning the game, but the complexity of it intrigued me—as well, of course, as the thought of winning.
>
> The initial stages of the game always went quite well. I accumulated the requisite number of properties, and managed always to get the $10 for winning a beauty contest. But there always came a point in the game when my brother would introduce a new rule! Over time I realized that the new rules my brother introduced came only when I was winning, were always to my disadvantage, and often seemed contradictory to the new rules from our last game! I learned that saying "yes" is not the only part of the game to which I needed to pay attention. If I wanted to play seriously, I needed to know the rules.
>
> Within a few years I developed a reputation in my family. Whenever we bought a new game, I was the one who went through the rules before we started to play. "C'mon, Mitch!" they'd say as I delayed the start of many a game on a holiday morning. "We'll learn how to play as we go! You're holding up the game!" But I was not deterred. For me, knowing the rules made the game more fun and decreased that gnawing feeling like I was missing something. Even when I lost (which was frequently), at least I knew that I gave the game my best shot.

The Basics

Informed consent and confidentiality are closely related—they are both crucial elements of our mansion's structural integrity. Psychotherapy is different from virtually all other relationships in which clients participate. The rules are not intuitive. Thus, informed consent involves giving your clients information about the rules of the relationship, including the parameters of confidentiality. You also provide information about you as a psychotherapist: how you work with people who are dealing with the issues they are facing, your training, and the nature of the therapy you will be doing. This information is critically important for prospective clients to know before they say "Yes, I want us to work together."

There is evidence that therapists do not implement informed consent as well or as often as they might (Dsubanko-Obermayr & Baumann, 2010; Trachsel et al., 2015). Talking through the "rules" of the relationship can be difficult, partly because they can seem too counterintuitive to clients—and to us! It is also difficult because several tripping points may converge. For example, if we know a client was in therapy before, the label ("anchor") of "previous client" might lead us to overestimate their familiarity with the information we are providing. Thus, we may not check their understanding as well as we should. We may employ the confirmation bias by interpreting their head nods or smiles as evidence of understanding or agreement (This might be especially true for clients of different cultural backgrounds.). As we strive to make our fee structure and policies for missed appointments clear, the financial frame of our discussion may overshadow the ethical frame. Thus, we may pay less attention than we should to our client's right to refuse treatment. We may employ the substitution principle when we ask ourselves the easy question, "Did the client sign my form?" rather than the more difficult question, "Did the client understand what we discussed and make a truly voluntary and informed decision?" As icing on the cake, we may not notice any of these tripping points because of our bias blind spots.

Good informed consent may be the issue that makes the uniqueness of the therapy relationship most clear. Here's what we mean: Friends don't usually tell each other, "Listen, there's somebody on the next street that is a different kind of friend than I—perhaps you would do better with that person." Salespeople are not really obligated to tell customers that another store has a similar item that can do the job better. But in psychotherapy, therapists are obligated to tell prospective clients not only about their own therapeutic approach—risks as well as benefits—but also about other forms of help that the client may want to purchase. In the words of the ACA (2014) Ethics Code, Section A.2.a., "Clients have the freedom to choose whether to enter into or remain in a counseling relationship and need adequate information about the counseling process and the counselor."

What information do we need to give to clients? Let's take a look at two ethics codes that provide a good overview:

- NASW, 2017, #1.03: Social workers should use clear and understandable language to inform clients of the purpose of the services, risks related to the services, limits to services because of the requirements of a third-party payer, relevant costs, reasonable alternatives, clients' right to refuse or withdraw consent, and the time frame covered by the consent. Social workers should provide clients with an opportunity to ask questions.
- ACA, 2014, #A.2.b: Counselors explicitly explain to clients the nature of all services provided. They inform clients about issues such as, but not limited to, the following: the purposes, goals, techniques, procedures, limitations,

potential risks, and benefits of services; the counselor's qualifications, credentials, relevant experience, and approach to counseling; continuation of services upon the incapacitation or death of a counselor; the role of technology; and other pertinent information.

Think back to Mitch's story of playing Monopoly with his older brother. Some of you might have thought, "No big deal. It's just a game." You might be competitive yourself and winning is very important. For you, it seems reasonable for Mitch's brother to gain an advantage by hiding or fabricating some of the rules. Others of you might have thought, "Well, that was a crummy thing for Mitch's brother to do! What about the value of playing fair—even in a board game!" Another group of you might think, "Even after going over the rules, does he really understand the game?"

In therapy, there is no debate about being fair or about the inappropriateness of hiding rules from clients. The therapy relationship is a collaborative relationship that is built upon trust. You facilitate trust when you help clients understand the rules and they can make reasonable decisions about therapy with you.

Journal Entry: *Informed Consent in Our Cultures of Origin*

Part 1: Consider your college experience. Most courses have a syllabus in which the instructor outlines the "rules" for the course and other important information. In the courses you took (are taking), think about the range of information you received on the syllabi at the beginning of the term.

- How did you react to syllabi that only provided a list of dates and assignments, versus those syllabi that contained detailed information about the course, such as course goals and prerequisites?
- To the extent you wanted information, why did you want it?
- Have you had a professor change the syllabus on you? How did that feel?
- Did you find that some syllabi were easier to read than others? If so, why?
- How might the syllabi have influenced your decisions to stay in the course, to take another course from the same professor, and to get more or less involved in the course than you would have otherwise?

Part 2: Think about some doctor visits that you have had or will have, especially when you go to the doctor for something other than a routine checkup.

- What do you want to know?
- How would you like to be told?
- What would it mean for the doctor to:
  - tell you the benefits of the treatment they are proposing?
  - tell you the risks involved? (What might NOT work in addition to what might work and how you might be worse off if you choose the proposed treatment.)
  - tell you about other options available to help with your problem?
  - remind you of this information at various times during the course of treatment?

If the doctor did tell you about the options:

- How well did you feel like you understood the options you had?
- How comfortable did you feel with the doctor to
  - ask questions,
  - ask follow-up questions if you didn't quite understand, and
  - refuse the treatment being offered?

The Three-Legged Stool

We refer to the informed consent process as a three-legged stool. An interesting property of three-legged stools is their stability—they do not wobble! A good informed consent process provides a stable foundation for psychotherapy. The three "legs" on which informed consent rests are ethical, legal, and clinical. These three aspects of informed consent influence each other as we work with clients.

Ethical

The most common ethical justification for the informed consent process is that it respects clients' autonomy (Foundation #3 in Table 4.1; Fisher & Oransky, 2008). Clients have a right to information, with which they become better consumers of professional services. Professional relationships of any kind work better when professionals and clients share some of the decision making—which means sharing information.

Informed consent is also a way to avoid harm to clients (nonmaleficence, Foundation #2; Crawford et al., 2016) and to maximize the benefits of treatment (beneficence, Foundation #1; Lambert & Barley, 2002). Knowing the rules often helps us win the game! By assuring client access to good information, informed consent procedures help therapists actualize fairness and social justice by minimizing disadvantages some clients experience due to differences in educational levels, cultural background, level of familiarity with psychotherapy, and other factors (Foundations #4 and #5).

In addition to these very direct justifications, there are several indirect ethical benefits. By clearly defining the professional relationship in an informed consent process, therapists are helping define and maintain boundaries. By thinking about what information to provide to clients and by considering the risks and benefits of their own and others' forms of psychotherapy, therapists are helping to maintain their competence. They may also avoid some of the tripping points we mentioned earlier, as well as the red flags of "Everybody's Everything" and "Dissing the Different." Indeed, they are exhibiting the green flags of "Amicable Advice About Alternatives," "Responsible Referrals," "Informative Information," "Guarded Guarantees," and "Effective Ethical Explanations." If they take their informed consent responsibilities seriously, they are actualizing and enhancing their professional virtues such as honesty, humility, and prudence (Foundation #8).

Legal

The ethical justifications for informed consent are complemented by legal requirements about who can and cannot give consent, what kinds of information needs to be conveyed, and how much information is enough. States have laws about who can and cannot give consent. For example, children up to a certain age (which varies by state) and legally adjudicated incompetent adults cannot give legal consent to psychotherapy. Some states require therapists to disclose certain information at the outset of psychotherapy so that clients know what they are consenting to. In addition, some states require psychotherapists to provide information in a written "disclosure statement." Typically the required information is about the psychotherapist's training and some of the laws that influence the practice. For example, in Colorado psychotherapists are required to inform clients in their disclosure statement that, "in a professional relationship, sexual intimacy is never appropriate and should be reported to the board ..." (CRS 12-43-214, 2016). A detailed description of legal requirements is beyond the scope of this book (see Appelbaum & Gutheil, 2019; Barnett et al., 2007).

Some therapists might be tempted to ignore their legal requirements, reasoning that if they take care of the ethical requirements they have done more than enough. This would be evidence of a separation strategy. Other therapists, perhaps adopting an assimilation strategy, might have their attorneys write their consent documents for them and ignore the ethical doctrine. An integration strategy, of course, includes both ethical sensitivity and knowledge of the law, as well as consultation with colleagues and attorneys.

Clinical

Until now you might have the impression that the requirements of informed consent represent a foreign appendage to the therapy process—a necessary but cumbersome requirement to get out of the way before therapy begins. Not so. Informed consent is an important part of the clinical work. Starting the therapy relationship with good information about the "rules" and respecting the client's right to refuse treatment provides a useful foundation for the working relationship (e.g., Birch, 1990; Coyne & Widiger, 1978; Jensen et al., 1989), and ensuring that the client truly understands what they are being informed about might actually increase the level of trust clients have for therapists (e.g., Handelsman, 2001a; Sullivan et al., 1993). At the same time, there is wide agreement in the field that we should view consent as a *process* that happens throughout therapy, not just an *event* that occurs at the beginning (Appelbaum & Gutheil, 2019). "Informed consent is an ongoing part of the counseling process, and counselors appropriately document discussions of informed consent throughout the counseling relationship" (ACA, 2014, Section A.2.a.). It is useful to think of clients consenting to treatment every time they come to a session. The process model of informed consent can stimulate and facilitate the clinical course of therapy. For example, information about the process of therapy may stimulate clients to think about the goals of therapy, and the consent can be renewed—officially or implicitly—whenever the goals of therapy evolve.

   The good news is that by looking carefully at the intersection of clinical, legal, and ethical concerns, we can explore many aspects of our professional identity. At the same time, however, issues surrounding consent can cause many types of acculturation stress and tripping points. Let's take a closer look now at the elements of informed consent.

The Culture of Consent

It is easy to say that we will give all of our clients all the information they need to make a good or informed choice about whether to see us in therapy. However, just as we learned in the last chapter about confidentiality, informed consent is multifaceted and difficult to achieve in practice. Several motivations, values, and virtues come into play as we meet with new clients and help them assess the client–therapist fit.

Motivations and Virtues

Let's start with a journal entry to get you into the acculturation mood.

Journal Entry: *Personal Components of Informed Consent*

Take a look back to Chapter 1 and the activities you completed about your needs, motivations, values, and virtues. How do these elements of your identity, your core, mesh with the justifications for informed consent we mentioned in the previous section? Do you see any situations in which you might feel a small yet strong urge to dispute or override a client's initial refusal to enter therapy with you? What situational or contextual factors might increase that feeling? What information might you want to hide or share less about so that clients are more willing to work with you?

When you think about the different types of information you'll need to share during the informed consent process, write down some about the feelings and reactions you might have with a client who (a) is a different race or ethnicity from you, (b) is a different gender or gender identity from you, (c) is one you find very attractive, (d) appears very anxious, (e) appears very depressed, (f) has difficulty speaking English or your native language, or (g) is in some other way challenging to you.

Food for Thought: *Getting Along with a Long Consent Process*

Consider this scenario: You are seeing a new client, telling him all about your therapeutic approach and about the alternatives he may want to consider. The client seems unsure, and begins to ask lots of questions about the therapy, about you, and about other types of treatment. You cannot tell whether the client has a genuine interest in these topics or he is just "messing" with you. You find yourself getting frustrated and you wish he would either sign the consent to treatment form or just leave. What tripping points might you be dealing with? What do you do? What is happening to your motivations? Are they becoming a little more varied, a little more cloudy? How does the virtue of patience interact with the other virtues that you have identified as important to you as a therapist? What might happen when you get in touch with your core?

Here's another scenario we'd like you to write about.

Journal Entry: *Informed Refusal*

Picture this: You go through an informed consent procedure with a client, explaining all the risks and benefits of your treatment and those of other treatments. You do a very informative job. (Think through what you would say—how you would phrase what you can offer, etc.) You know you can help the client. You are very enthusiastic. As you listen to yourself you think, "Wow, I have lots of excitement in my voice. I would love to work with this client and I think I am explaining my expertise well."

At the end, the client thanks you for such a clear explanation. Then she says, "Thanks, but no thanks. I'm going to pursue other options." She mentions one of the alternate treatments that you discussed, but you know the treatment is longer and perhaps less likely to work.

- How do you feel? Are you disappointed? Are you angry, frustrated, or irritated? Do you feel like a failure?
- What do you want to say to the client?
- Are you tempted to suggest other benefits of your approach or other risks of the others?
- Can you respect the client's autonomy? What would make it easier to do so and what would make it harder?
- What alternatives do you have? What acculturation strategies might those alternatives represent? What alternatives might be evidence of the substitution principle, ethical fading, or other tripping points?

When clients choose to go elsewhere—especially one who has visited with us for an hour or two—it might at least hurt our professional pride. An experience like this can also disturb our professional myths about being helpful or about being the right therapist for every client. This type of experience may be especially hurtful when our emotional defenses are low, such as when we're experiencing problems in our personal relationships or financial problems are looming.

- Consider some complicating factors, such as:
  - You need the clinical hours to graduate on time.
  - You need the billable hours and you know money is no object for this client.
- What virtues would you like to exhibit and in what quantities?

Perspective Taking:

- You have a friend who makes a similar choice not to enter therapy with a psychotherapist you think would be good, and asks your opinion of their decision. How do you react to your friend? What's the difference between your reactions to your client and to your friend?
- You are a client meeting a therapist for the first time. The therapist gives you a very informative picture of the benefits and risks of her approach and others. As good as the presentation is, you find there's something that doesn't "click" for you with this therapist. One of the alternative approaches she mentions is new to you and sounds very interesting. You decide you'd like to give it a try. You say, "Thanks, but no thanks. I'm going to explore other options." How would you like the therapist to respond? What do you imagine is going through their head?

Not-So-Simple Consent

In the example above, a client refuses treatment. A refusal makes it clear that the client does not want to work with the psychotherapist and shouldn't be forced. True consent is voluntary (Appelbaum & Gutheil, 2019). However, in some instances the client is not voluntarily in therapy. For example, when a court orders a person to undergo treatment, the court is exercising its right to act in what it believes is the client's welfare. This is an example of paternalism; the court's judgment about the client's welfare overrides client autonomy. Indeed, one could argue that a person under the auspices of a court does not even have autonomy to be overridden.

Another example of more complicated consent is when people are not capable of giving consent because they are not cognitively able or competent to understand enough about the situation to make a reasoned decision. One example of this is young children who are brought to treatment (either individual or family) by parents or guardians. Another example is adults who are suffering from mental disabilities. Sometimes they are adjudicated (found by a court) to be unable to give consent. Psychotherapists recognize that when clients cannot give consent they are still worthy of respect and deserve to be informed about what is happening in a way they can understand. In these cases, therapists should get *consent* from parents or guardians and *assent* from the client. Several ethics codes (e.g., ACA, 2014; APA, 2017) require psychotherapists to seek assent, which means "to demonstrate agreement, when a person is otherwise not capable or competent to give formal consent (e.g., informed consent) to a counseling service or plan" (ACA, 2014, p. 20).

The application of assent may seem counterintuitive. Try this food for thought.

Food for Thought: *Assent*

Part 1

Picture this: You are a child therapist and the parents bring a 12-year-old boy for you to see. You believe you can help, the family is very motivated, but the boy is refusing to give his assent—his permission. On one hand, you'd like to honor his wish not to come. On the other hand, both you and the parents agree that even though the boy doesn't want to come, you believe you can make therapeutic progress with him.

To give you some perspective on what this might feel like for the 12-year-old boy, consider an experience you may have had in a security line at the airport. You've finished going through the security door and your briefcase or backpack comes out the other side of the scanning machine. The security agent at the station says, "May I examine the contents of your backpack?" The security person is asking for your *assent*. You can perceive this request in two ways, sometimes depending on how much of a hurry you are in: First, you can see the request as nonsensical. Why would you ask that question when only one answer is acceptable? After all, if you don't give assent to searching your backpack you'll have to stay home or leave your backpack at the airport. Second, you can see the request as a courtesy—one step up from "Have a nice day." You and the agent both understand the situation you are in. Neither of you really enjoys the process but both are constrained to be there. Given that, you are both respectful as you "go through the motions."

Part 2

Consider the options you have when a client refuses to give assent. (a) You can choose not to see the client. In this case, you may not have made any progress, but you may miss the chance to do some good work. (b) You can see the client in spite of their non-assent. Here, you are reversing the risks of the first option. (c) You can explore the consequences of the non-assent. Clients may not have considered the probabilities of losing services, going to jail, or continuing to be miserable with their parents. (d) You can try to compromise, perhaps having the client assent for three sessions and then reevaluate.

For each of these options, think about your core (and other) motivations, acculturation stresses, and tripping points as you work with court-ordered clients and child clients, some of whom you like and some of whom you do not.

Is it just going through the motions to seek assent in therapy? Perhaps not. Some clients may not give permission and you assess that they will probably not benefit from the services you are providing. As a result, you choose not to see them. In that case, you would consult with the parents, a guardian, or the court. But don't make the "rookie mistake" of thinking that just because a court- or parent-ordered client expresses the desire not to be in therapy, nothing can be done. Good work can happen under less-than-ideal conditions. You will likely choose to see some clients who do not give you permission, and in all of these cases it is respectful to ask the client to assent to therapy and inform him or her about what will be happening.

Information: How Much, of What Kind, Presented in What Way, Is Enough?

How do we know that a client has enough information to make a good choice about therapy without being overwhelmed by it? The question of what is enough information—and other questions surrounding informed consent—is an example of how much complexity there is behind the straightforward standard that we provide informed consent (Wise, 2007).

When dealing with informed consent in medicine, most courts adopt a *reasonable person* standard (Murray, 2012) when determining how much information is enough. The question is: What would a reasonable person want to know about therapy? In Appendix A we list the types of information you might want to (or have to) disclose. We list some key areas that help clients know more about the therapeutic process, the logistics of therapy, the therapeutic process, ethical issues, and you and your training.

Green Flag: *Informative Information*

Marian and Clara have come to a therapist, Dr. Shaw. They are having some problems with their daughter, Ashley, and these problems are either a cause or an effect of some of their marital problems. They're not sure whether they want to come as a couple, or simply to send Ashley to a therapist. After describing some of the problems, Clara asks Dr. Shaw, "So tell me, Doctor: What experience do you have with issues like ours?"

Dr. Shaw responds, "I've had training and experience with couples, and if you want to come in for marital work I'd be happy to see you. But it's been a long time since I've seen adolescents for individual therapy, so I wouldn't feel comfortable seeing Ashley. Sometimes, it's good for a kid of Ashley's age to have her own therapist and not see her parent's therapist, anyway. If you decide to send Ashley to a therapist, I can certainly give you some names of therapists who specialize in working with adolescents."

Food for Thought: *Persuasive Information*

Think about the major approaches to therapy you have studied, including psycho-dynamic therapy, cognitive-behavior therapy, family therapy, existential psycho-therapy, and so forth. For each approach: How would you describe that type of therapy to a friend of yours who may benefit from that approach, but who has not studied psychotherapy at all? Take two approaches. Can you think of ways to describe each approach that would make your friend more interested in either of them? Can you think of ways to describe each approach that would be more neutral, or even make your friend less likely to choose either of them?

Journal Entry: *Information, Please*

Spend some time writing about the following questions:

- What information do you *need* to convey to all clients? This information could be mandated by law, required by an ethics code or agency policy, or so basic to your work that you believe every client should know it before agreeing to see you.
- What information might you let clients know they have a right to ask about (Pomerantz & Handelsman, 2004)?
- What information might you want clients to know because it will help the therapeutic process?
- On the other side of the coin, what information might you not share with clients because you believe it might actually get in the way of good work (Beahrs & Gutheil, 2001)?
- What information will you disclose if asked, but only if clients bring it up? This information might be personal and/or irrelevant to therapy.
- What information would you not tell clients even if they ask?

- What questions might a client ask that you know would bring great discomfort? How would you deal with that discomfort?
- How do you think questions by clients need to be answered and in what format (e.g., oral, written)?
- How would you know if the client really understood the information you provided them?

How we inform clients may be related to our core—the values and virtues we hold. Providing information to clients in writing is a good idea (Handelsman, 2001a), and some states require written disclosure. An even more positive approach is to give clients a copy of the consent form (Nagy, 2000), as it increases the likelihood that clients will remember and be able to use information.

The APA (2017) code requires that we document the informed consent process. Once again, we have several types of judgments to make, including this one:

Food for Thought: *Perspective Taking on Documentation*

Let's explore some different levels of specificity in documenting consent. Let's say you are (a) a therapist, (b) a member of an ethics committee that is investigating a therapist who is alleged to have made "guarantees of success," or (c) a new intern who is taking over a therapy case from an intern who has graduated and left the agency. What level of specificity (written information) would you (a) do, (b) be looking for, and/or (c) appreciate?

- "Client signed the consent form."
- "Client and I discussed aspects of the treatment."
- "We reviewed the consent form. Client asked about the limits of confidentiality, and didn't understand at first about what 'danger to others' meant. I provided some examples of specific threats that would be reportable. Client was somewhat relieved that I wasn't going to report him just for being angry. When he signed the form, he asked for a copy before I even offered him one, and I told him that we'd go over all the information again in 5 weeks. In all the things we discussed, client seemed most concerned about the risks of treatment I outlined—becoming more depressed, disruption in relationships, etc. Perhaps his being anxious about these things happening is related to the clinical picture of someone who is hesitant to take risks, not confident in his ability to follow through on projects, and somewhat pessimistic."

Acculturation Tasks and Stresses

As we mentioned before, conveying information and securing consent in psychotherapy are not analogous to many other types of relationships. Thus, part of the experience may be very uncomfortable for many therapists. Sometimes it is hard to see the informed consent process as part of the treatment process, especially when the discussion turns to risks, ethical issues, and personal information.

We love to talk about the benefits, but we may be more hesitant when it comes to discussing the risks of treatment and alternative treatments. How do you feel about talking about what might go wrong? Some psychotherapists might think that talking about risks undermines the therapeutic process. Actually, predicting that rough spots are likely to come with change might have a much better effect on the therapeutic process. Remember, many clients are coming in already anxious and are likely to feel unconvinced by a message like, "Everything will be fine and therapy will be smooth sailing."

Red and Green Flags

Consider the following responses from four different therapists. We'll leave it to you to identify the flags—to give you some practice.

> Darnell, 46, is facing anxieties that some people would call "midlife issues." His wife, Maria, seems more demanding and less sexually receptive now that their nest is empty. Their son, Darnell Jr., is struggling financially to make ends meet and Darnell senior is worried about that. At the first session with a therapist, Darnell describes these anxieties and says, "I am not even sure about being here but my brother-in-law who is in school said I should check out a cognitive approach because it works really well for these kinds of things. I'm a cognitive kind of guy. I'd really like that."

Dr. Weeve

Dr. Weeve says: "Look, that cognitive stuff doesn't work for everybody. I think what you need is a caring, compassionate therapist, and that's what I do. I've been doing that forever. I've had lots of clients like you, who come in wanting a cognitive approach and they're merely avoiding getting to the root of their existence. What they needed is what you need: a good active listener. And that's me. In fact, I had one client just about your age, who had been a high school teacher and decided to go back to school for a MBA and work in stocks. Well, that was right around the tech stock bust, so he stopped that and …"

At this point, Darnell is wondering why he's getting all this detail. He thinks, "I know people who used to be high school teachers; is she describing somebody I know? And why is she bad-mouthing a style of therapy my brother-in-law, Trevon, thinks is effective?"

"… did very well. In fact, I'm seeing him on Thursday afternoons."

Darnell says, "Thank you, Dr. Weeve. I'll think it over." Yeah, right.

Dr. Kidder

"Well, that kind of approach is pretty easy. I've taken some courses on it. I'm sure we can do that. Let's give it a try." As he leaves the office quickly, Darnell thinks to himself, "I wonder how much training a therapist needs to be good, or even adequate, for this kind of therapy. I need to ask Trevon." He decides to keep looking.

Dr. Tully

"I agree with you—for cognitively oriented people, it can be really great. But I'm afraid that's not my area of training. I've had a few courses, but no supervised experience. Let me give you some names of colleagues who do this kind of cognitive work."

Dr. Haive

"I see you're referred by Dr. Tall; I know him. Yeah, cognitive therapy is one of my areas of expertise. Let me tell you more about what I do with clients in this approach and I am also curious about why you think your brother-in-law thinks this might be helpful. After we talk, if this sounds right for you and you sense we'd work together well, then we'll proceed. If not, I can give you names of other cognitive therapists with whom you might work better."

To give you a sense of some stresses and tripping points, consider this: Picture a psychotherapist, during their first session with a client, feeling uncomfortable about discussing ethical issues. Their discomfort might produce this thought: "If I bring these things up I'm just putting ideas into their head to see me as unethical." The therapist may simply want to avoid some annoyance and get on with the good work of therapy. They may not realize the tripping points or red flags that might appear quickly. For example, they might decide not to bother with the details of limits to confidentiality. Their thinking might be, "Look, if I go into an oration of limits of confidentiality—about reporting child abuse and needing to protect the target of a serious threat—I am going to dissuade the client from feeling free to share anything with me. I think I am just gonna let the conversations go until I think there might be something where I need to let them know." Or the therapist might be uncomfortable with questions about experience working with people from a different ethnic background or social identities and gives a cursory response.

At a minimum, this therapist is not demonstrating the green flag of "Informative Information." For example, clients have a right to know the limits of confidentiality from the start and the therapist's experience with people who look like them. The therapist may not be recognizing that conveying information about any issues with care—ethical issues, experiences with diverse populations, risks, etc.—may enhance the therapeutic process even though it may take some time.

Our impatient/anxious therapist may be one step away from various additional problems. They may be thinking, "This client doesn't speak English well, and is hard to understand. This could take a long time, and the chances of these situations coming up is so small." Now, we have the red flag of "Overlooked Oppression": It might be hard for our therapist to spot, but making a decision based on language or avoiding questions related to diversity might be evidence of a pattern of infringing or denying rights based on issues of difference or racism. The language issue or the client's concern about experience may override the therapist's good thinking. We can see ethical fading: The convenience and/or financial frames have taken over at the expense of ethical and/or cultural ones (green flag: "Cultural Cognizance").

It is easy for the therapist to rationalize the decision not to disclose information about limits to confidentiality: "We've gotten to the substance of therapy quicker— I've saved the client money!" "I'm a good listener; therefore, my therapy will be good for the client (self-serving attribution)." "I'm increasing access to treatment!" "Look, the client is opening up to me. (confirmation bias?)" These may sound good at the time. But please consider one more variation on the scenario: In the third session, the client shares information that can't stay confidential and now the therapist has to backtrack and discuss confidentiality. Trust is now a big issue for the client. He or she has the right to wonder, "What else has my therapist not told me?"

The deliberations and rationalizations that sounded so good in the therapist's head do not sound so good now. The decision not to provide information to which all clients are entitled or answer questions that clients have legitimate concerns about was not a wise one and compromises the relationship.

Have we painted a picture of an unethical, dastardly, racist therapist? No. We have no labels at all for this therapist, other than "human." We have portrayed a person who is making some very bad judgments and is not mindful. Think of it this way: When we make decisions like this we are losing touch with the fact that we are in the mansion and that every room (the confidentiality, informed consent, and issues of diversity rooms) in the mansion is important. Although our intentions might be good, we are all prone to such lack of awareness of our tendencies, biases, tripping points, and red flags. Such a lack can last for a few seconds (which is long enough to make bad decisions) or it may be a lasting pattern.

Journal Entry: *Credentials*

Questions about your degrees and licenses may seem like clients' idle curiosity, but actually have a lot to do with the ethical issue of competence and with the relationship you form with your clients. Think about the following questions:

- How do (will) you feel when clients ask you about why you are qualified to see them? Are you or will you be hesitant to answer such questions?
- How do you feel about clients who ask you questions that seem challenging or overly detailed?
- What if a client asks you for the complaint procedures of your state board?
- How will you communicate your credentials? Big diplomas on the wall? Or will you list memberships in professional organizations, even though they are not really indicators of competence?

The answers to these questions may give you some insight about your motivations, values, and virtues.

Now, let's to one step further: Go back to Chapter 4 and look at the tripping points and flags. Go back to Chapter 3 and look at the acculturation strategies. With these in front of you, we want to encourage you to explore deeper, more complex questions that possibly push past bias blind spots.

See our questions below:

- If I were using a separation or assimilation strategy, what will my responses look like to the last set of questions? To which strategy will I lean when not at my best?
- How will I respond differently (worse) if I ignore the clients' cultural or other backgrounds?
- To which three tripping points will I be *most* prone? Financial pressures? Avoidance of ambiguity? Ethical fading?
- What aspects of my core identity will I be the first to lose touch with when under stress? How will that manifest itself in shifting my decisions and actions? What green flags will not be there and what red flags will emerge?
- How will I incorporate the green flags of "Privilege Perception" and "Common Consultation" (and others?) into my thinking and acting?

Notice that we use the word "will" in these question, rather than "might" or "would." Are we saying that you are unethical? Of course not. That would be making the Fundamental Attribution Error. We are simply encouraging you to realize that we are all capable of small lapses that have big implications. We want to get you into the habit of honest self-reflection.

Perhaps the most acculturation stress and opportunities to trip come from clients asking personal questions. Personal questions come in all shapes and sizes, ranging from those with professional aspects to very private questions. We might be tempted to respond fully to all requests for personal information—after all, complete honesty is a virtue, is it not? Remember in Chapter 5 we talked about boundaries. Depending on various issues such as context and client identities, we need to temper honesty with other virtues, such as prudence and compassion.

In our striving to avoid ambiguity and achieve simplicity, we might be tempted to have a policy of "no answers to personal questions." This might be evidence of an assimilation strategy. It is too absolute and may not give you the flexibility to make decisions based on the type of information requested, the needs of clients, their cultural identification, your core identity, and other aspects of the situation.

One good strategy for dealing with such questions is to consider every personal question from a client as a potential boundary crossing (see Chapter 5, especially the section on self-disclosure). Think about issues such as beneficence (Foundation #1), review the questions in the last journal entry (e.g., concerning cultural issues, tripping points), and judge whether the answer to the questions will help the client and build more trust in the therapy relationship.

Developing integration strategies in response to personal questions will include balancing issues such as awareness, honesty, prudence, beneficence, and respect. It may mean responding to clients' questions in creative ways. For example: Lew and Toshiko are seeing Dr. Haive for marital therapy. Just after the small talk at the first session, Lew asks with an air of politeness but perhaps an undertone of challenge: "So, are you married?" Dr. Haive replies first with a simple "Yes" or "No." She then follows up with something like the following to explore the concern behind the question: "I'm wondering if you have concerns about whether I'm qualified to do couples therapy with you both?" Toshiko immediately says, "Of course we think you can!"—but with a worried look. Lew is thinking, "Damn right, I'm concerned!" but says out loud, "Well, now that you mention it …"

Another therapist might respond to the question about marriage this way: "I'm wondering whether you want to know if I've been through the kinds of problems you are going through." This response is reasonable because it shows that you are aware that all clients' questions have substance to them. Curiosity may be idle, but clients and their questions are not! By inviting the client to explore that substance, you make it clear that your own personal experience is not the only, or the most basic, issue.

When Mitch was a young therapist, one question he would ask clients was, "How many couples would it take for me to have seen before you would feel comfortable?" This question made it easy to start talking through their concerns about his competence. It also provided Mitch with the opening to make it clear that the only way to see whether he could help them is to give him a few sessions and then reassess their comfort level.

Another important acculturation task brought up by the informed consent process is to decide how collaborative the decisions about therapy are. What kind of power do clients have? Some information you provide to clients is to educate them so they can make the decision to enter therapy or not. Clearly, they have the ultimate power and authority to make that decision. However, some information will allow clients to make other decisions that you may have thought were entirely yours. For example, you and the client may collaborate on decisions about how long to stay in therapy, what kinds of strategies (of those in which you are qualified) you will use, and how the client will be involved in treatment.

We end this chapter with a green flag story. As you read through the story, try to identify all the green flags you believe Dr. Verdi demonstrates.

Green Flag Story

Belle and Scott were upset and nervous when they came to the first session with their new therapist, Dr. Kelly Verdi. After all, this was the first therapy experience either of them had ever had. Belle was feeling unsupported and wondering whether Scott may be having an affair. Scott was exasperated and felt railroaded into therapy. They were both concerned about their daughter and her weird new friends at school.

Belle and Scott were both thinking that they'd better get the first word in before their spouse contaminated Dr. Verdi's judgment with false information. If they could only explain their point of view, each of them thought, Dr. Verdi would surely just tell the other what they needed to do to solve the problem.

Imagine their surprise when Dr. Verdi didn't let either of them speak! The first thing she did was give each of them what seemed like a stack of papers. "I know this may not be what you're expecting, but I want to begin our therapy with some clear ground rules. Let's go through the major rules together, shall we?"

Dr. Verdi explained that she typically sees both members of a couple but at times may want to see one individual if she thought it would help. Belle asked, "What if Scott tells you something in secret? Are you going to keep that from me?" Dr. Verdi explained that she would not keep secrets if those secrets were getting in the way of the couple treatment.

"What if I choose not to come?" Scott said, a little more angrily than he meant.

"You always have the option to terminate therapy, Scott," Dr. Verdi said evenly. "Even if you decide to come for several weeks and then decide this isn't for you, you have the right to stop treatment."

"Would you still be my therapist if Scott decides he doesn't want to come in?"

Dr. Verdi smiles, glad that this issue came up so soon. "We all need to talk about what your goals are, both individually and as a couple. It might be better if I work with both of you on the issues that have a direct influence on the relationship. But if you want to work on some things individually, it might be a good idea for one or both of you to work with a different therapist on your own."

Belle asked, "We think our daughter may need some help; can you see her?"

"If it will help me get a sense of the family and your relationship, it might be that I'd want to see your daughter. But teenagers need somebody to talk with privately, and she may not want to open up with her parents' therapist. Again, she might do better with her own therapist."

Belle continued: "Wouldn't her therapist tell us what she was discussing?"

Dr. Verdi responded, "Different therapists have different policies. When I see an adolescent in therapy I discuss with everybody, at the beginning, what kinds of information I'll convey to the parents. Usually, because I believe that kids need some privacy, I'll ask the parents to agree that I only share information when there's a clear risk to the safety of the kid."

Scott chimed in, "But the parents are paying!"

"That's right," Dr. Verdi said, "and legally they have a right to the therapy information about their kid. But I ask parents to waive that right so that the kid can get the most out of therapy."

The questions and answers went on for most of that first session. There seemed to be more and more options about therapy and Belle and Scott were undecided about what to do. But Dr. Verdi was in no hurry for them to make a commitment. "You need to think over what we've discussed and look over the other information I've given you," she said. "You can contact me if you decide to come in and we'll set up an appointment. If you choose not to see me, I'd be happy to give you names of other therapists who might be helpful."

At the end of the session, Belle and Scott got up slowly, as if they were both weighed down by the volume of information they had gotten and the enormity of the decisions they needed to make. But they agreed on the drive home that they felt good about Dr. Verdi because she had answers to all their questions, as if she had thought about them beforehand. And she didn't pressure them to make a quick decision. "At least we know what we're getting into," Scott said.

"Yeah," said Belle. "Some of that stuff about us seeing other therapists would have come as quite a shock if we were three months into treatment. It's good to know this stuff now."

"Maybe we should see her for three or four sessions. Then we can have another one of these sessions where we make a final decision about who sees whom for what."

"I agree," said Belle. "That's a good idea." It was the first thing they agreed on all week.

8

Making the Most of Supervision

Sharon starts this chapter by sharing the following supervision experience that occurred during her doctoral internship. Check out the food for thought activity that follows her story.

> There I was, with tears starting to form, telling my internship supervisor about my confusion in a current romantic relationship. Penny sat there listening with ears picking up on my every word and eyes intently watching my nonverbal cues. As I leaned back in my chair I thought, "How did we get onto this topic?" I remembered talking about the clients I was seeing, especially those with whom I was having some difficulty. Then I started to share some about my career goals and job application process. At that point, my thoughts got fuzzy and I began to talk about me, the person down deep inside who was trying to make sense of a conflicting personal situation. As my emotions began to unravel before Penny, she—in her gentle yet candid way—asked questions, reflected back my feelings and words, and provided some options for me to consider. Later, as I left her office and walked down the hallway to mine, I felt both clearer in my thoughts and ready for my next client of the day—one of the very clients with whom I was having trouble.

Food for Thought: *That Was Some Good ...*

How would you finish the sentence above?

- a) That was some good supervision!
- b) That was some good therapy and supervision!
- c) That was some good therapy, but it should have been supervision!
- d) That was some good ____ (you fill in the blank)

In a couple of sentences, explain why you finished the sentence the way you did.

The Nature of Supervision

Supervision is a professional necessity—it is a service to the profession and the public in which a more experienced professional takes on the task of training and monitoring a less experienced professional. Bernard and Goodyear (2019) define supervision as "an intervention provided by a more senior member of a profession to a more junior colleague or colleagues who typically (but not always) are members of that same profession" (p. 9).

Ethical and effective supervision doesn't just happen—it takes knowledge, skill, and diligence. Supervision is a specialty that requires training to develop a unique combination of "knowledge, skills, and sensitivities" (Maki & Bernard, 2007, p. 347) in areas including psychotherapy, training, and student development (Stoltenberg & Delworth, 1987). A professional can be an ethical and effective clinician yet not a good clinical supervisor. Thus, some states now require people who want to be supervisors to take special training and secure specific credentialing in clinical supervision.

Supervisory relationships may provoke some of the most common and acute acculturation stresses and tripping points for both supervisors and supervisees. After all, there is no more universal "rite of passage" for psychotherapists than supervision (Maki & Bernard, 2007), which has been described as "the critical teaching method" (Holloway, 1992, p. 177) in the helping professions. Here's the way Bernard and Goodyear (2019) described the nature and sometimes conflicting goals of supervision:

> This relationship is evaluative and hierarchical, extends over time, and has the simultaneous purposes of enhancing the professional functioning of the more junior person(s); monitoring the quality of professional services offered to the clients that she, he, or they see; and serving as a gatekeeper for the particular profession the supervisee seeks to enter. (p. 9)

More than once we have told our students that supervision in practicum and internship can make or break the experience of entering the profession. Before we look in detail at ethical issues inherent in supervision, let's explore who you are at your core when it comes to being given direction and/or receiving feedback.

Food for Thought: *Authority Figuring*

Think about some times when you have been evaluated (in a non-job situation) or have needed help from somebody else regarding some skill. These times might be about tennis lessons, learning a musical instrument, or submitting drafts of your master's thesis to your advisor. They can include any time when you were facing somebody who was acknowledged as more expert than you and had some type of authority over you. As you think about these instances, we ask you to explore the following questions:

1. When advisors, teachers, golf pros, and other authorities make suggestions about what to do, what are your initial emotional reactions? Anger? Gratitude? Embarrassment? Joy? Sadness? (How did it feel to be behind the wheel when there was a big "Student Driver" sign on the car?)
2. When somebody points out a flaw in your performance, how do you react? (Did you react to this question by saying to yourself that you've never had a flaw to be pointed out?)
3. Do you like to learn on your own or are you quick to ask for assistance? (How quickly, if at all, do you ask for directions when you are lost?)
4. When learning to master a skill, how important is it for you to appear competent even as you are learning? (When offered assistance, how quick are you to respond, "That's OK, I can do it.")

Take some time to think about your responses. Is there anything that surprises you? What did you notice about your attitude when learning something new, when asking or not asking for assistance or instruction, and when receiving either positive or critical feedback?

The Ethical Complexity of Supervision

The content and context of supervision is intricately bound up with ethics; the passing on of experience and expertise is central to the development of a "competent practitioner" (Corey et al., 2007, p. 350). Rather than simply review the rules around ethical supervision, we want to take a more comprehensive and positive approach. Our starting point is to recognize the complex roles of both supervisors and supervisees.

Supervisors are ethically and legally responsible for their supervisees' choices and behaviors (Harrar et al., 1990). They must continually balance the needs of many people and entities, including trainees, clients, agencies, state regulatory bodies, and their own selves. These are significant obligations and a prime example of possible acculturation stress and tripping points for supervisors. For example: Because of the multiple frames involved—training, client welfare, time commitments, financial considerations, gatekeeping functions—supervisors may be at risk for ethical fading. Because of the intensity of the relationship, supervisors may be prone to the affect heuristic and subject to the confirmation bias when they evaluate supervisees.

On the other side of the relationship, supervisees have their own stresses and balancing acts. Supervisors expect supervisees to enter into the relationship with a willingness to be vulnerable about their strengths and challenges as therapists. However, in previous relationships (e.g., with professors), students have been reinforced for being, and for appearing, strong and perfectly competent. Thus, supervisees face the new tasks involved in balancing their interests in appearing competent to their supervisor with being humble and honest so they can learn a new set of skills. They need to embrace supervision that both supports and challenges them. Thus, for both supervisors and supervisees, engaging in supervision is itself an act of moral courage!

Haynes et al. (2003) highlight the ethical and legal responsibilities for supervisors in terms of four supervision goals: (a) facilitating professional development; (b) protecting client wellbeing; (c) assessing the supervisee's competence and, if need be, preventing supervisees from entering the profession; and (d) helping supervisees become adept at assessing their own skill level and performance. To help both supervisors and supervisees, we add four ethics-related goals for supervisors to attend to: (a) maintaining boundaries within supervision; (b) establishing an informed consent process in supervision, (c) addressing value differences between supervisor/supervisee and supervisee/client and exploring their impact on both supervision and therapy, and (d) acknowledging supervisees' cultural and social identities.

At this point, let's dig a little deeper into the acculturation process by building upon the Food for Thought: Authority Figuring.

Journal Entry: *Acculturation to Supervision—The Good, the Bad, and the Beautiful*

Think of a time when you were supervised in a job or task. It could be with a psychotherapy supervisor or any kind of structured job or professional supervision. Now that you have that in your mind, write down your responses to the following questions:

1. What are some things that happened in the supervision that prompted you to grow and develop?
2. What are some things that happened in the supervision that hindered you from growing and developing?
3. How did you contribute to the good outcomes?
4. How did you contribute to the bad outcomes?

5. If you erred in some way, how? Was it wanting to do things your own way, not taking enough initiative and simply doing what you were told, just doing the minimum required, and/or something else?
6. If your supervisor erred in some way, how? Was it micromanaging your work, not providing enough feedback, not connecting with you, and/or something else?

Sherry (1991) discusses three factors that make supervision difficult and supervisors "vulnerable to misconduct" (p. 568). The first is balancing competing role obligations, the second is that the supervision hour can feel "therapy-like," and the third is the power differential between supervisors and supervisees. To explore the first factor, we present two food for thought activities for you that highlight competing obligations in supervision.

Food for Thought: *Your Favorite Student*

Imagine that you are on the part-time faculty of a training program and that part of your work is being a supervisor. Sue, one of your favorite supervisees, is just finishing her practicum before going on internship. Late in the semester during one of your supervision sessions, Sue casually mentions that she happened to run into one of her clients at a coffee shop and they visited for a little while. With a bit more information, you find out this wasn't really an accidental meeting but something that was scheduled. When you ask how long this has been going on, she says, "I've only done this once or twice with a few of my clients whom I feel benefit from the more informal interactions."

"Why haven't you told me this before?" you ask.

"It's not like a date or that I'm having sex with these clients; it's always been in the interest of the therapy. It actually seemed to be helping our work in therapy and I didn't think it was important to mention it."

From your view, Sue has not only stumbled on some tripping points, but she has violated some ethical standards. Although you still have some information to get, you believe Sue's actions are grounds for a dismissal hearing in front of the program faculty and ethics committee. If Sue is found guilty of unethical behavior (which she surely would be), the faculty and ethics committee have several options: They could discharge her from the program, delay her internship for a year, fail her in her practicum, or put a letter of admonition in her file. How do you react?

- Do you let the program faculty know and file the case with the ethics committee?
- Do you have a "heart to heart" conversation with Sue, letting her know that what she has done is serious enough to warrant an ethics committee investigation?
- Do you consider her stellar academic record and decide to let this go if she promises to tell you absolutely everything she's doing in therapy from now on?
- What tripping points might be operative in your deliberations?

You check the program handbook, and the policy clearly states that "all ethical infractions by students need to come to the attention of the program." As you're thinking this over, consider the following questions. Which of these are you most tempted to think or say?

1. "I know it's program policy, but this can be handled much more effectively in the context of our supervision. I am not going to turn this into a big deal."
2. "I've got to turn this into the program faculty and ethics committee. What will they think of me if I don't?"
3. "This program is too rule-based. Students make mistakes but are not unethical people. After all, I've been Sue's supervisor for a while and I know her better than the ethics committee."
4. "This is an uncomfortable situation. I really value Sue's work and she's done a good job. This misstep is serious, though. I think I need to bring this up with the faculty and discuss our possible courses of action."

Which acculturation strategies might each of these statements represent? Which tripping points might make you lean toward one strategy over another?

Your reappointment for working as part-time faculty the following year is not certain. You wonder how this particular issue with Sue might influence your future in the program. What variables might influence your decision about whether to share the details with the faculty and ethics committee or deal with the issue yourself?

5. How would your reactions change under the following conditions?
   A. Sue was an international student from Kenya.
   B. It was Sue's first semester in the program, rather than last.
   C. Sue was not one of your favorite supervisees; in fact, the two of you never really connected.
   D. Sue asked you to keep this from her major professor, who would "have my behind" if he found out.
   E. Sue was Sam.
   F. Sue had only gone for coffee once, with one client, after she had successfully terminated therapy.
   G. Upon further investigation you find that she only went for coffee with clients who were attractive and single.

Food for Thought: *Your Favorite Supervisor*

Put yourself in the place of a trainee. You are talking to one of your fellow trainees about a particularly difficult and distasteful client. You inadvertently mention his name. Your colleague says, "Are you serious? That's my cousin!" You apologize profusely to your colleague, and extract from her a promise not to turn you in for your breach of ethics, assuring her that you will tell your clinical supervisor.

As your meeting with the supervisor looms closer and closer, your thoughts wander to several different options. First, you consider the possibility that it would be respectful to your client if you told him about the breach of confidentiality and apologize to him. You wonder what your supervisor (whom you really like and trust) would say about that. Then you think, no harm was actually done to the client and he doesn't need to know of the breach. And then there is the good impression you have been making on your supervisor recently and the letter of recommendation she has promised to write for you.

1. Consider the following possible steps:
   A. You choose to tell your supervisor about your behavior. Why?
   B. You choose **not** to tell your supervisor about your behavior. Why?
2. How do your reasons fit with the values and virtues in your journal entries?

Now, imagine that you do tell your supervisor, who thinks it over and then says to you, "What you just told me is an ethical infraction. I'm afraid I need to inform the rest of the clinical staff and the program's ethics committee. I am not sure what the consequences will be." Which of the following is closest to your reaction?

1. "I deserve to be kicked out of the program. That was an unacceptable ethical error."
2. "I made a mistake. I'll address the clinical staff and ethics committee as best as I can and learn from the situation. I'll ask for a second chance."
3. "Slipping up and mentioning a client's name is not that big of a deal. I am sure my supervisor has done it. They are being way too harsh."

Which acculturation strategies might these statements represent?

Think about what facts would need to change for your reactions—and your acculturation strategies—to be different.

Role Obligations and Informed Consent

As supervisors, we try to balance the need to provide a supportive atmosphere, which is conducive to good supervision (Carifio & Hess, 1987; Martino, 2001; Wulf & Nelson, 2000), with our gatekeeping role—keeping some trainees out of the profession. We try to achieve this balance by being very clear about our goals with supervisees. For example, in Sharon's ethics class and then in the teaching/supervising practicum, she addresses this balancing act when she shares two very important messages with her students. The first message is that supervision is characterized by concurrent and appropriate levels of support and challenge. The support part is about Sharon providing an environment where supervisees experience a safe place to be honest, humble, and accountable about their work with clients. Sharon knows that when supervisors create a safe supervision relationship, supervisees can feel freer to share their work openly and more effectively (Barnett et al., 2007). When the safe space is in place, supervisees can seek and accept critical feedback and develop the ability to benefit from increasing levels of challenge.

The challenge part is about carefully assessing supervisees' skill level and ability–ensuring that their clients are receiving the best possible service. Sharon's goal is that clients receive good counseling while the trainees continue to grow and develop as competent, ethical counselors.

Sharon's second message to her students and supervisees may be perceived either as a harsh reality or as a shared superordinate value: Although she cares about her trainees and their professional development, she makes it clear that her greater obligation of care is for their clients. If her assessment is that supervisees are harming clients and are unable or unwilling to make the necessary changes to improve their craft, she will prevent those supervisees from entering the profession. For example, if a supervisee is impaired and clients are not being well served, it is her ethical obligation—to the client, the supervisee, and the profession—to address the issue.

Sharing this type of information is part of the informed consent process in supervision—the first of our four ethics-related goals. Similar to informed consent with clients, it is important that the supervisor and supervisee enter into an informed consent process (Bernard & Goodyear, 2014). It helps to think of the relationship as a contractual one (Sherry, 1991) in which expectations, obligations, and other issues are clear from the outset (e.g., Barnett & Molson, 2014; Bernard & Goodyear, 2019; Borders et al., 2014).

Bernard and Goodyear (2014) suggest that the following information be included in the informed consent document: roles and obligations of the supervisee and supervisor, goals for supervisee and supervision time, policies and procedures to be followed, parameters around confidentiality, competencies to be obtained, evaluation processes and criteria, and grievance procedures.

One advantage of an explicit contract is that it might help both supervisees and supervisors assess their fit with each other. Another advantage is that supervisees will know their performance requirements early on. A third advantage is that supervisors may be clearer—with themselves as well as their supervisees—about their philosophy of supervision. A final advantage is that logistical issues—such as financial arrangements and emergency procedures—can be anticipated and clarified.

Food for Thought: *Informed Consent and Supervision*

Look back to Chapter 7 and consider the parallels between informed consent in supervision and therapy. From the supervisee's perspective, ask yourself: What other information would you like to know about supervision and your supervisor? Then, from the supervisor's perspective, ask yourself: What would you want a supervisee to know before they choose to work with you?

The Therapy-Like Feel of Supervision: Boundary Issues and Beyond

Our second goal is to maintain boundaries in supervision, so that the other supervision goals remain front and center. Supervision is—or at least appears to be—similar to psychotherapy in some ways: One person comes to another for help; the professional relationship is key to the success of the enterprise; and there is power to be used, shared, and potentially exploited. But there is one major difference: For therapists, the concern for clients' welfare is paramount. Therapists are concerned with the person in the room with them. In supervision, however, the *ultimate* concern is the welfare of the supervisee's clients—who are not in the room—even though supervisors have clear obligations to facilitate supervisees' development.

A second difference is that supervisees have ethical obligations in a supervisory and therapeutic relationship that clients do not have in the professional relationship. For example, supervisees need to be honest, self-reflective, prudent, and humble with their supervisor. Supervisees also have obligations to their clients to be competent, truthful, and concerned about client welfare. Clients, on the other hand, aren't obligated to demonstrate these same attributes.

One typical phenomenon in supervision is *parallel process*, in which something is happening in supervision that is similar—in an important way—to what is happening in therapy between the supervisee and client. For example, there have been times when our supervisees felt frustrated with us when we've asked questions (rather than gave answers), which is strikingly similar to the client's response when our supervisee asks questions rather than giving answers to the client. In each case, the person frustrated just wants "the answers."

Another common manifestation of parallel process concerns *countertransference*. At times, a supervisee will connect or react too strongly with something that is transpiring in the client's life. The client is no longer just the client; they are or feel like someone else to the supervisee. This countertransference can be happening, at the same time, between a supervisor and supervisee; the supervisor's perception is skewed. When this happens, objectivity in roles can be or is lost, and the risks include negative outcomes and disrespect to both clients and supervisees (McNamara et al., 2017).

Understanding parallel process can give us insight not only into our clients' behaviors, but also into our own behaviors, motivations, and needs as both supervisors and supervisees. This takes us back to the opening story of the chapter:

Food for Thought: *Therapy or Supervision?*

In response to the story that Sharon shared at the beginning of the chapter, how did you finish the sentence: "That was some good ...''? With that in mind, consider the following questions:

1. What was your first impression of what occurred? Did it sound like supervision or did is sound like therapy?
2. What else would you want to know to answer Question 1 more definitively? In other words, what distinguishes therapy from supervision?
3. As a supervisor, how much personal information might you want to know about your supervisee's life to know how you might best help them develop?
4. As a supervisee, what type of questions from your supervisor might you find helpful and wish to answer?
5. On the other side, what type of questions from your supervisor might you find intrusive and think you should not have to answer?
6. Have you had a similar experience in a supervision session? If so, what did it feel like to you?
7. Reflect on the different issues we've explored thus far and see which ones relate to Penny (the supervisor) and which ones relate to Sharon (the supervisee).

The sometimes fluid boundary between therapy and supervision brings up other boundary considerations. Think about the issues we discussed in Chapter 5; many of them can be applied here. Consider, for example, the supervisor who engages in inappropriate self-disclosure during supervision sessions, or brings their personal problems into the sessions, or shows bias or discrimination against supervisees based on supervisee's personal beliefs or lifestyle (Cornish et al., 2008). In a parallel way, think about a *supervisee* who engages in inappropriate self-disclosure (during therapy or supervision), brings their personal problems into sessions, or shows bias or discrimination against clients—or against the supervisor.

Negotiating boundaries might be more difficult in supervision than in therapy because the differences between supervisees and supervisors may be less salient than those between clients and therapists or students and professors. For example, both supervisees and supervisors are professionals in the same field, they are both there to discuss the problems of the client, and they might be closer in age than the client and supervisee. Thus, the illusion might be that boundaries can be more fluid in supervision. However, we take a similar position as in Chapter 5 regarding boundaries between therapists and clients: We believe that keeping boundaries as free as possible from competing obligations and conflicts of interest serves everyone best. As Beddoe (2017) noted, "The best interests of supervisees are served by supervision in which boundaries are maintained, the relationship is respectful, and the focus is primarily on professional development" (p. 91).

Food for Thought: *Boundaries*

Scenario 1

Sarah, a first-year professor in the graduate program, thought that her supervision with a first-year student, Arturo, had been unusually intense but unusually productive. Arturo was the first person in his family to go to college, let alone graduate school. Many of the supervision sessions consisted primarily of Sarah sharing her "wisdom" about academia with him; after all, she had landed this plum job only six months ago. In these sessions, Arturo had talked a lot about his own feelings of intimidation and his fears of not doing well. Arturo had done well with his clients and asked that Sarah be his supervisor for the next semester. Sarah accepted the invitation and looked forward to working with Arturo again.

One day while she and Arturo are talking in her office, Sarah gets the call she'd been waiting for: a summer position at a research lab on the coast! She tells Arturo, who shares her excitement. Before Sarah realizes what she is doing, she asks Arturo, "Would you like to house-sit my house this summer?"

Scenario 2

Susan appreciated the way Krisann worked with clients, especially children. On several occasions Krisann found a way to connect with even the most reserved and reticent child. For sure, Krisann was one of the best psychotherapists-in-training that Susan had worked with. Krisann was graduating in the summer and Susan was pleased to write a letter of recommendation.

At their last supervision session for the term, Susan and Krisann briefly shared their plans for the summer. When Krisann found out that Susan and her husband were taking a short vacation and needed child care, Krisann quickly volunteered, "I would love to babysit your kids!" At first, Susan felt relief. She believed Krisann would be a great and trustworthy sitter for her children. And of the few sitters she trusted and typically employed, none of them were available for that long weekend. But then Susan started to feel uneasy. She felt like this could be a problem of role confusion. So, she said, "Thanks for the offer Krisann, but I think it's probably best if I don't hire a student to babysit my children."

Look back to Chapter 5 and respond to the following questions:

1. Are there potential boundary crossings or violations in these situations?
2. Do any of the green flags or red flags apply here? If so, which ones, and how?
3. If you were Arturo or Krisann, what would you be thinking? What tripping points might influence your thinking?
4. If you were another student who heard about this offer from Sarah to Arturo or the offer from Krisann to Susan, what would you be thinking?
5. What factors or changes in the scenarios might make the situation either more or less serious?
6. If you were on an ethics committee and were considering a complaint against Sarah in Scenario 1, what might you be thinking?

Power Differential

Although the differences in roles between supervisor and supervisee sometimes seem much less salient than those in other professional relationships, the stakes are very high and the power dynamics are complex. Much of the power derives from the evaluation and gatekeeper roles supervisors play. Of course, properly balanced and judiciously applied power can be of benefit—indeed, is essential—to both supervisees and their clients. However, research reveals that supervisors can use their power in very harmful ways. Ellis (2017) gathered stories from trainees who experienced horrible treatment by their supervisors and lack of accountability by the agency or organization that employed their supervisors. Ellis's research revealed experiences where supervisors' abuse of power included racism, sexism, ageism, and no informed consent process or written contract.

Another misuse of power in supervision is indoctrination. By this we primarily mean that supervisors squelch supervisees' professional growth by limiting their ways of working with clients only to how the supervisors would do it. This would be parallel to therapists advising clients to solve problems the way the therapists have, even though clients have other resources to use.

Another type of indoctrination is related to personal values. Supervisors may impose their personal values within supervision that, in turn, influence supervisees' work with clients. Regarding issues such as abortion, drug use, and politics, for example, supervisors might encourage trainees to hold values and/or nudge their clients in a particular direction that matches the supervisors' values. This is clearly an ethical misstep and parallel to the supervisee trying to impose their values on the client. In terms of conflicts of values between the supervisor and supervisee, McCarthy Veach et al. (2012) suggest that unaddressed value conflicts within the supervision relationship result in negative impact on supervisee development and client services.

Hence, our third goal for supervisors is to attend to, rather than ignore, value differences or conflicts between the supervisee and client as well as those between the supervisee and the supervisor. Dunn et al. (2017) state, "Since it could be argued that no value is objectively and demonstrably wrong, then it would seem reasonable to conclude that supervisee and supervisor equally contribute to the value conflict and have responsibility to work toward a mutual resolution" (p. 205), with the onus being on the supervisor to address the conflict.

Dunn et al. provide a model for supervisor and supervisee to use when addressing differences in values. The takeaways from the model for our discussion are the following: Supervisors need to provide an environment where supervisees feel safe to discuss value differences, whether they be with the client or the supervisor. Supervisors need to normalize the conflict in values that supervisees experience, recognizing that they are part of the professional journey. Supervisors need to do their best to remind themselves and the supervisee that the client's welfare is the most important part of the resolution.

Our fourth goal for supervisors is acknowledging the supervisee's cultural and social identities. In Chapter 2 we discussed how important it is for therapists to acknowledge and honor the client's identities. This is no less true in supervision. Some of the harmful acts reported by Ellis (2017) were about supervisors debasing or minimizing the supervisee's identities. These acts were devastating and dehumanizing. Our cultural and social identities are a central piece of our core and in many ways can't be or shouldn't be cut off when we enter the therapy or supervision room. We bring our whole selves into the room; what we do with our whole self is critical. It seems duplicitous for supervisors to encourage and train their supervisees to see and work with their clients as whole persons and then turn around and not see and/or bring into the discussion the supervisees' whole self (social and cultural identities), encouraging supervisees to compartmentalize a part of themselves.

Making the Most of Supervision

The professional literature suggests that the relationship between the supervisor and supervisee is important (Barnett et al., 2007; Loganbill et al., 1983); even more important than the techniques and models/methods used in supervision by the supervisor (Inman et al., 2014; Kilminster & Jolly, 2000). A healthy, functional relationship is one free of power struggles and replete with healthy doses of virtues on the part of both parties. The supervisee needs to experience the supervisor as empathic, respectful, supportive, and committed to or emotionally invested in the supervisee's development (Kennard et al., 1987; Watkins, 1995). Both parties need to experience the other as trustworthy and collaborative in the relationship (Ellis, 1991; Henderson et al., 1999; Ladany et al., 1999; Wulf & Nelson, 2000).

Virtues

We see several virtues as being key to a productive supervision relationship. The first is honesty. Think back to what Sharon shares with her trainees about the client being the primary stakeholder in both the counseling and supervision relationships. Because the client's welfare is of utmost importance, supervisors need to give honest feedback about how supervisees are performing as psychotherapists. Likewise, supervisees need to give honest information about how therapy is progressing and how they are experiencing supervision.

Remember in Chapter 1 when Sharon shared her supervision experience? Her professional ego got pinched when her internship supervisor pointed out her missteps with a couple and even highlighted her colluding with the wife's verbal harshness in the relationship. Her supervisor's honesty did hurt, but because it was tempered with virtues like compassion it obviously had an impact, seeing as how she can remember the conversation so many years later. The second part of that story (and the part she likes to remember the most) is that in her next session she corrected the situation directly with the clients. She shared with them her supervisor's observation and apologized to the husband for not really hearing him. The therapeutic work then continued on a better track.

Honesty also refers to honesty with oneself. Supervisors need to be honest about their interests, their personal and professional reactions to supervisees, their motivations, their potential biases—and their mistakes. When honesty is a norm of the relationship, each party can be real and feedback can be more effective.

Being real and honest in the supervisory relationship overlaps with a second important virtue: humility. Supervisors need to be clear about the limits of their competence and not promise supervision in an area that goes beyond their scope of practice. Supervisees need to be willing to receive negative as well as positive feedback about their work and embrace the guidance given to make course corrections. And both supervisors and supervisees need to be willing to apologize for oversights, mistakes, or lost opportunities to have made supervision better.

Humor can be an important virtue in combination with humility and honesty. Being willing to laugh at yourself and sharing the humor in otherwise difficult situations are healthy dynamics in the supervisory relationship. They allow us to gain perspective. For example, when supervisors share their human foibles, supervisees can relax a bit and come to see that to be a "good therapist" does not translate into being a "perfect therapist."

This is only a partial list of necessary virtues. Look back to your own list and see how your virtues—the ones you have and the ones you need to develop—apply on both sides of the supervision relationship.

When Things Go Wrong

Unfortunately, it is not rare that some degree of conflict occurs in supervision (Baird, 1999). More recently, these times of conflict have been referred to as "supervision ruptures" (Watkins et al., 2019, p. 282). Reasons for such conflict include personality clashes, supervisory style, differences in theoretical orientation, neglect, lack of empathy or responsiveness, cultural differences, multicultural insensitivity, misunderstanding in role expectations, and cultural differences (Bernard & Goodyear, 2019; Ellis, 2017; Friedlander, 2015). When a rupture occurs there are several steps to take and issues to consider. De Golia and Corcoran (2019) offer the following acronym for supervisors to consider: O/D-WID-R and R, which translates to Observe/Detect-Wonder, Inquire, Discuss-Repair, and Resolve. When our intuition or supervision sixth sense kicks in that something is amiss, we need to use immediacy with empathy and ask the supervisee if we are detecting a shift in the relationship and if so, what that change might be for them, and if need be, use our humility and apologize to repair the relationship.

From the supervisee's perspective, it is important to see the conflict as an opportunity to learn something about yourself—look for that nugget of gold even when responsibility for the rupture is shared. Try to identify what the conflict is about—and it is seldom about only one thing. It is a good idea to get clear in your own mind how you see the conflict before you discuss it with your supervisor. Ask yourself, "What part of this conflict am I responsible for? What principles or virtues are at stake? How I am willing to change?" Then, try to see the issue from your supervisor's point of view if you can. Perspective taking is an important element in any human relationship.

As a supervisee you have a difficult problem on your hands when the supervision you are getting is poor and/or you are experiencing harm from the supervisor. The supervisor could be technically incompetent, temporarily impaired as a professional, and/or emotionally unstable. All or some of these may result in ethical lapses and not fulfilling their duties to you and your clients. Confronting a supervisor can be a difficult process that takes a large dose of moral courage. It may be necessary to seek out support and guidance from another professional, a faculty member at your program, your own therapist, and/or others. Sometimes it's hard to talk with other faculty members: We have seen students go through a whole semester of poor supervision, not saying anything to us or other faculty. The student's thinking was either, "I can't tell anybody because I'll be seen as a poor student," or, "I am probably just overreacting and I can get through this on my own." Students often suffer alone in bad supervision when at a minimum they could have shared their burden with other faculty members and likely have gotten some support.

A Word About Consultation

Although the skills and activities involved in consultation are similar to those in supervision, there are important differences. Here are two: First, consultation is between two peers, whereas supervision is between an experienced professional and a less experienced professional. Second, the consultant is expected to give good professional advice and direction to the person seeking consultation; however, there is no legal liability on the part of the consultant. In supervision, the supervisor is ethically and legally responsible for the professional practice and choices of the supervisee.

Here's an interesting reality that sometimes professionals realize too late: You'll never be too experienced or too much of an expert not to need some guidance! Consultation is a wonderful gift to give and receive—and sometimes it's a critical necessity. It is important to maximize the benefit you get from consultation; therefore, we have a few suggestions for you about how to choose a consultant.

Our first suggestion is to remain humble enough to ask for help when you need it. Second, consider whether you want clinical and/or ethics consultation. Although in both cases you want to look for experts, we feel that ethics consultation may take a little more prudence as you select a consultant. For example, when choosing a clinical supervisor you might want to find someone who is more expert than you in your own form of therapy. However, if you need ethics consultation, it might be more prudent to choose a consultant who is expert in ethics but who does *not* work with clients from the same theoretical orientation! This will give your discussions more perspective.

Third, do not consult with colleagues who are your friends! Again, this is especially true for ethics consultation—you do not want to put friends or close colleagues into the awkward position of having to give you bad news about your ethical behavior. They may not be as objective or forthcoming with you as you need. Choose someone who you trust, or at least think, will give you the straight story versus someone who will tell you what you want to hear.

Fourth, make consultation routine. Set up regular consultation with a group of professionals who commit to being honest with each other and call for accountability among the group members. Keep these people as professional relationships; stay away from the temptation to make them friends or part of your social group.

Finally, we feel that the more serious the problems you are having, either clinical or ethical, the more formal you want the consultation relationship to be (Gottlieb et al., 2013). This means you should begin the relationship with an informed consent process. Document the consultation. Pay for it. This will help you take it seriously and get the perspective and guidance you need.

Green Flag: *Beneficial Boundary Bolstering*

Dr. Newman hadn't been in practice long when she realized that the world is more complex than the academy! She knew all the platitudes about "Put your client's needs first," "Provide enough information so your clients can make good decisions," and "Don't exploit your clients financially." But putting these into practice with a wide range of clients was a daunting task. Dr. Newman decided to hire an ethics consultant who could look over what she was doing and suggest some ways to make what she considered an ethical practice even better.

The first person she thought of as a consultant was her old ethics teacher, Professor Sandoval. He knew her well, and he always told his students, "Let me know if you have questions."

When Prof. Sandoval heard from Dr. Newman, one of his best students of the last few years, he was delighted. It made his heart feel good to know that his students had learned the lessons he tried to teach, including the value of thinking about ethics and the ongoing nature of ethical development. When she asked to see him as a consultant, however, Prof. Sandoval needed to teach one more lesson.

"I'm not the person you want for this," he started.

"But … but … you said we could contact you with questions. You wrote that wonderful letter of recommendation for my internship and my first job! You said I was one of your best students."

"That's *exactly* why I'm not the best person to give you consultation. I'm biased, if only slightly, and my interests are conflicted. You remember when we talked about the confirmation bias? I may see your behavior as confirming my high opinion of you, and miss some red flags that others would see. You need a consultant who can be objective and honest. I think I could be honest, but it might be hard for me to tell you that what you are doing is not good."

"But I just need somebody to look at what I'm doing in case …" Dr. Newman trailed off, as if she started to realize just what Prof. Sandoval was about to say.

"Yeah, but think of a situation in which you get complained against," Professor Sandoval said, picking up on Dr. Newman's growing insight. "What would an ethics committee say when you told them that you got consultation from your old professor, a colleague who was already favorably predisposed toward you and might see your behavior as reflective of *his own* professional effectiveness? How objective is that going to look? I can give you names of a few folks whom you don't know who can offer you better service for what you need."

"I see what you mean," Dr. Newman replied. After she got the names from him and thanked him, she hung up the phone and immediately decided to increase her annual donation to her school's alumni association.

9

Ending Psychotherapy
The Good, the Bad, and the Ethical

"Parting is such sweet sorrow."
—Shakespeare

As we write this penultimate chapter, the end is in sight—in fact, we're facing a looming deadline. Here are our questions: When will we know that the book is good enough to publish—when is it actually finished? Do we have enough journal entries in each chapter? Does our discussion of boundaries lean too heavily on our own values, or not enough? Are we being too prescriptive in the chapter on informed consent? Have we been inclusive and sensitive to issues of culture, sexuality, oppression, and discrimination? Have we really gotten our important points across to help readers with their ethical acculturation? Did we explain well enough what we mean by your "core"? And because of our explanation and your exploration, do you have a better sense of who you are at your core and who you want to be in your profession? Have we provided adequate practical guidance? Are we positive enough in our approach?

When we think about our effort and own competence we wonder: How do we know when we have put in enough effort, with enough impact, to produce an optimal outcome? At what point is a sub-standard product so bad that we are displaying incompetence? At what point would more polishing of the manuscript be evidence of our own fear rather than our desire, and ethical obligation, to help our readers? We can never have perfect answers to these types of questions; we would need *infinite* time and *infinite* judgment. However, if we used this lack of perfection as an excuse and ignored these types of questions, the manuscript may turn out to be of little value.

In therapy, the same types of questions arise: "How do we know therapy is over?" "Have we done all that we can for now?" "Are we ready to say 'goodbye'?" However, you might be saying to yourself: Why is there an entire chapter on termination? The questions about ending therapy are much easier because I have the client right there. All I need to do is ask.

Most ethics books don't emphasize the issue of termination; however, several ethics codes declare the importance of this part of therapy. For example:

- AAMFT, 2015, #1.9: "Marriage and family therapists continue therapeutic relationships only so long as it is reasonably clear that clients are benefiting from the relationship."
- NASW, 2017, #1.17(a): "Social workers should terminate services to clients and professional relationships with them when such services and relationships are no longer required or no longer serve the clients' needs or interests."
- ACA, 2014, #A.11.c. "Appropriate Termination: Counselors terminate a counseling relationship when it becomes reasonably apparent that the client no longer needs assistance, is not likely to benefit, or is being harmed by continued counseling."

These guidelines seem to be straightforward and to the point. Seems pretty simple—all we need to add is the idea that clients are free to terminate and we're covered, right?

Almost! The basic principles of termination—the client has the choice of when to terminate, therapists should terminate when therapy isn't working any more—are not so easy to implement, for two reasons. First, these two principles often conflict with each other. Second, terminations involve difficult clinical judgments in a variety of contexts, complex personal reactions and tripping points, and challenge many of our virtues. Here's a related example: When we finish writing this book, we will feel elated, relieved, and probably quite successful. Years of hard work will have paid off, our professional identities as educators will have been bolstered, and our values of achievement and industry will have been actualized. However, we will experience other reactions as well: We will feel concerned that we've missed something, or that we could have anticipated the needs of a wider spectrum of our readers. We will feel sad to lose the opportunity to work with each other. We may even feel scared at having to face the void left by the completion of our task—what do we do now?

In a similar way, psychotherapy termination always means a complex set of cognitive and emotional reactions that relate to your ethical core and acculturation. Let us begin our exploration with some self-exploration.

Journal Entry: *Endings*

How are you at ending relationships? What do you experience in these endings and how do you navigate them? Think about several different types of relationships you've had that have ended, including (but not limited to) some of the following:

- romantic relationships;
- close friendships that ended when you graduated or moved away;

- roommates;
- relationships with co-workers, employers, or employees.

Think about relationships that have ended because (a) you initiated the ending (breakup, move, etc.), (b) the other person initiated the ending, and/or (c) the ending came about because of external circumstances. Think about endings that were good and those that weren't so good. Think about endings that you've regretted. Now, reflect in writing on these questions:

- How did (do) you feel at the end of these relationships?
- What is your typical pattern with ending relationships before they need to be ended? For example, are you more likely to quit before you get fired, leave before you get dumped, or do you hang on to the relationship even when the "writing is on the wall"? To what extent does a sense of loyalty influence your decisions to continue or end relationships?
- What types of endings to what types of relationships are relatively easy for you?
- When endings are difficult, to what extent do you look for internal guidance (go with your feelings), and to what extent do you look for external sources of help (e.g., saying things like, "Our policy is such that …")?
- Do you "walk away," perhaps just to end the uncertainty, or are you the type of person who likes to "process" the end—to look back and reflect on what the ending means?
- How else might you characterize what you think, feel, and do at the end of different types of relationships?

The Good and the Ethical: Positive Elements of Termination

Ending psychotherapy is complex and includes a combination of ethical, clinical, and practical variables that interact with each other (Davis, 2008; Davis & Younggren, 2009; O'Donohue & Cucciare, 2008). One positive way to think about termination is that it is the logical conclusion to the ongoing informed consent process that occurs during therapy. It may be the time that the client, with full information, finally chooses to say, "I'm done." Indeed, some authors have encouraged therapists to discuss termination during the initial consent process (Davis & Younggren, 2009; Kramer, 1986). Rice and Follette (2003) advise therapists to "take responsibility at the beginning of a therapy contract for educating the client on how the termination process will unfold and what criteria you will be using to evaluate their progress" (p. 157). All relationships end; explicitly acknowledging this fact at the beginning of a therapeutic relationship provides useful information for both therapists and clients. Davis (2008) suggests several competencies necessary for successful endings across a multitude of situations. Therapists need a solid ethical foundation, self-awareness, relationship skills, clinical assessment, case conceptualization, understanding clients' expected experience of termination, and cultural influences.

Both the APA (2017) and ACA (2014) codes mention *pretermination counseling*. For example, the ACA code states that "counselors provide pretermination counseling and recommend other service providers when necessary" (2014, A.11.c.). Pretermination counseling provides information so clients can make an informed refusal and, similarly to the informed consent process at the beginning of therapy, get information about other sources of help. Even when therapy ends well, you and your client can take some time to recap your work and the therapeutic relationship, talk some about how it feels, and say goodbye. Of course, sometimes clients drop out of therapy before any pretermination counseling can be done.

We'll talk later about how you might provide some pretermination information in the most ethical way. For now, we turn our attention to some difficult ethical decisions you will face in every therapeutic relationship you have. We've organized this discussion around two practical questions. They will help you navigate the ethical landscape and integrate your needs, motivations, values, and virtues from your ethical cultures of origin, the tendencies about endings that you identified in your journal entry, and professional standards and principles. The questions revolve around when should therapy end and who decides.

When Should Psychotherapy End?

The best-case scenario is when you and your client agree on when therapy is over. Sometimes, however, you and the client have different ideas about whether this is the end, and sometimes the answer isn't even clear to you. We assume that the decision about when therapy is over can be very emotional for clients. We need also to remember that it can be emotional for us because it involves our core values, professional identities, clinical judgment, and therapeutic orientation.

Let's assume for the moment that there is an objectively and determinable perfect time for any therapy to end. At the risk of sounding like Goldilocks, we can look at termination along a continuum: it can be too soon, too late, or just right. When we say "too soon" or "too late," we are not talking about a matter of minutes, hours, or days; even weeks might still be within ethical limits. After all, physicians are not always sure of the exact time when a cast should come off or a medication be discontinued. At some point, however, rushing or delaying termination goes beyond acceptable judgment, perhaps beyond poor judgment. It can move to a situation in which clients do not benefit as much as they could have or in which they are harmed.

The ethical components of deciding when therapy is over include: having the clinical competence to assess progress or the lack of progress of therapy, and the virtues of prudence and humility which allow us to make determinations without our personal needs getting involved and to actualize our professional values regarding such issues as what therapy is for and what it means for particular clients.

One condition under the "just right" part of the continuum is for all the client's presenting problems to be solved. Another condition is that the results of the therapy are *good enough*. In these scenarios, not all the client's problems have been solved, but enough have been resolved so that the client feels ready—at least for some period of time—to walk through life without your guidance and support. A third condition is that therapy did not work well enough to continue. A fourth condition is that therapy didn't work at all, and a fifth that therapy actually harmed the client.

Food for Thought: *Is Therapy Over?*

Take a look at the following vignettes and ask yourself if these are satisfactory outcomes and whether therapy should end. Why or why not? Think of each vignette from the perspectives of (a) the therapist, (b) the client, and (c) a supervisor. Think about what you would do, or what you would encourage a supervisee to do—and why—from an ethical perspective. Think about how your response speaks from your core. Also consider what might be evidence of acculturation strategies of integration, assimilation, and separation.

- A client comes in to stop smoking and 7 weeks later has kicked the habit. However, now he's feeling some sadness.
- A woman comes in feeling depressed. Seven months later she is feeling much better—taking much more control of her life. She still reports times of sadness that last for long periods, but she is able to go about her life; e.g., she always manages to get to work.
- A couple comes in for counseling and their stated goal is to save the relationship. After 14 long months they agree to stay together. From your perspective it seems like one partner is getting the "better deal" and is more comfortable with the outcome than the other.
- A couple comes in for counseling. Their goal was to try to keep the relationship together—for the sake of the kids. After 14 stormy months they decide to divorce. Neither partner is happy, but they seem resigned to their decision and they both talk about looking forward to what the future brings.

Who Initiates the Discussion of Termination?

Let's expand our discussion by adding another dimension to the mix—who decides to end treatment, or who initiates the discussion. Figure 9.1 is our complete graphic showing both continua.

Clients can initiate a discussion of termination—or, of course, they can simply leave and not come back. Therapists can initiate the discussion and in some cases unilaterally decide to end treatment. Or the termination can be a truly collaborative effort. The best-case scenario is the latter, where both you and your client feel like the contract has been met. Alternatively, both you and your client may agree that therapy has *not* been helpful and is not likely to be. In either situation there is a perfect intersection of beneficence and client autonomy: what's best for the client in your judgment is also what the client is choosing.

Sometimes either the therapist or client initiates a termination discussion because of situational factors that impinge on clinical ones. For example, the therapist may be leaving an internship, or retiring. A client may be moving, or may lose their ability to pay, and need to transition to another therapist.

Relatively few therapies end right at the middle of our diagram. We are more likely to find ourselves in one of the other boxes, which represent unclear or conflicting answers to the questions of providing benefit and respecting client choice. Let's explore the top row first, in which therapists initiate termination.

Therapist-Initiated Termination That's Just Right

In spite of the adage that clients are in control of the decision to come for therapy, there are times when therapists need to initiate termination to uphold ethical obligations (Davis & Younggren, 2009). At these times, considerations of beneficence and/or nonmaleficence may override the client's autonomy. In fact, ethics codes discuss the need to terminate treatment if therapy is not helping or might be harmful, even when clients might express a desire to stay in therapy (more on this situation later). The obligation is to terminate a treatment that is not working and refer clients to

When To Terminate

		Too Soon	Just Right	Too Late
	Primarily the Therapist	[abandonment]		
Who Decides?	Both Therapist and Client		[perfection!]	
	Primarily the Client			[dependence]

Figure 9.1 A Matrix for Termination Decisions.

sources of help that may be more effective. One possible acculturation stress occurs when our personal feelings of care and helpfulness come into conflict with our professional judgment that we cannot provide what some clients need.

Therapist-Initiated Termination That's Too Soon or Too Late

Some therapists, with some clients, with some problems, may seek to terminate therapy too soon or too late. Why do you think this might be the case? Speculate a bit, using your knowledge of tripping points, virtues, acculturation, and other information. As you speculate, we invite you to reflect back on your journal entry from earlier in this chapter. Based on what you wrote, consider reasons why *you* may terminate too soon or too late. If you think you will be making (or do make) perfect choices with all the clients you see—think again.

One reason therapists may initiate non-optimal terminations might be predilections based on theoretical orientation. For example, at one end of the continuum are therapeutic approaches that encourage a thorough understanding of clients' personalities and comprehensive changes in many areas of client functioning. Therapists on this end of the continuum may be a little too hesitant to end therapy. On the other end of the continuum are therapy approaches that work on very specific problems. When the client overcomes the specific fear, for example, therapy is over. If clients have other issues they can sign up for another course of treatment with the current therapist or another therapist.

Differences in judgment about when to terminate based on therapeutic orientation may reflect legitimate differences in approach. When clients have been well informed, it is not unethical to have therapy be somewhat longer or shorter than it would have been with another therapist. However, when these theoretical predilections become biases and override other concerns and values, therapists may be at risk of violating competence, beneficence, and other guides.

Another reason therapists may not terminate at an optimal time is differences in ethical reasoning; for example, achieving the difficult balance between actualizing the principles of autonomy and beneficence. Some therapists may give autonomy a little more weight and allow clients to make decisions about termination that are not the best. Here, clients may derive more benefit from a little closer guidance by the therapist. Other therapists, perhaps using an assimilation strategy, might feel that their judgment of when to terminate—because it's so well informed by expertise— should be forcefully presented and accepted. Once again, reasonable people can hold different ethical theories. We believe, of course, that these theories are most useful when therapists apply them in the context of virtues such as humility.

Another reason therapists may not end therapy at an optimal time is their own feelings, including their sense of completion, achievement, and helpfulness. Some people like small achievements in incremental stages. Other people like to look at achievements on a grander scale. Think of it this way: Some writers write limericks and celebrate the completion of each one, others write short stories, and still others do not feel like writers until they complete an epic novel.

Therapists' decisions to terminate too early may exemplify the substitution principle. Complex questions may include the following: "Do I have bad feelings about this client or the therapy that may hinder further treatment?" "What will it take to finally make some progress with this client?" "Am I competent to enter a new phase of treatment?" Therapists may avoid these questions by asking a simpler one: "Is this an ok time to terminate the treatment?"

As you look back on your journal entry, see if you can become more aware of your own tendencies to say "goodbye" either too soon or too late. These tendencies could reflect personal issues, such as commitment or the need to be a helper; personal feelings like guilt or achievement; or tendencies based on ethically relevant dimensions. Also, we invite you to think back to your own ethics autobiography and the values exercises you completed in Chapter 1. How do you see your role as a therapist? Are you a life-long guide? Or maybe a short-term consultant? Think about yourself related to the analogy about writing and types of writing. Which seems to fit you? How would you adjust your need for completion, achievement, and helpfulness when it comes to ending therapy? What do you believe clients and you should get out of a successful therapy process? How might the answers to these questions influence your thoughts about termination?

Too Soon

Stopping treatment too soon might be considered *abandonment*, which several professional ethics codes specifically prohibit. For example, the ACA Code (2014, A.12) states: "Counselors do not abandon or neglect clients in counseling. Counselors assist in making appropriate arrangements for the continuation of treatment, when necessary, during interruptions such as vacations, illness, and following termination."

As we mentioned earlier, sometimes stopping therapy too soon is stimulated or influenced by external factors: the insurance money runs out, one party is moving, or the therapist is retiring or changing positions. But sometimes there are internal reasons—the therapist may have some unresolved countertransference, such as feelings of anger, boredom, or disgust. These feelings, of course, are a good indication that some consultation is necessary.

Too Late

The upper right box of Figure 9.1 represents cases in which therapists initiate termination too late. Therapists may terminate too late for a variety of reasons, including incompetence, external pressures such as the financial benefit, internal issues like the need to be needed and a lack of prudence or humility in relationship to other virtues such as diligence, or the combination of internal and external pressures involved in conflicts of interest.

Sometimes therapists make a technical mistake and don't realize either that the client's needs have been met or will not be met by the current therapy. Thus, the therapist wants to continue therapy longer than is wise. Therapists may even convince clients who want to terminate that they should "hang in there." Of course, this is ethically problematic and will likely result in harm rather than good.

Red Flag: *Sideline Solicitations*

Jenna has really appreciated the time her therapist, Dr. Pak, has taken to explain lots of different things she could do to improve her condition. They've talked about hiking, nutrition, yoga, some more hiking, taking classes at the local community college, a little bit more about hiking, tai chi, and—you guessed it—hiking. One day while waiting to see Dr. Pak, Jenna notices a new table in the waiting room. On it is a cardboard display with several copies of a book, *Hiking Trails in the Tri-State Area*. Jenna has to squint to see it, but she's stunned as she notices the author's name: Dr. F. Pak. Alongside the books are several types of energy bars. She picks one up and reads part of the label: "Pack some energy for your hike with Pak's Energy Packs!"

Now Jenna feels a little strange. She can't help but wonder whether the hiking recommendation came from good professional judgment or was just a set-up. She puts the bar down on the table and finds the energy to hike out of Dr. Pak's office and over to the State Board.

As you consider this case, don't be fooled into thinking that Dr. Pak's behavior is so extreme that it couldn't apply to you. Sometimes our better judgment can be compromised. We have other topics that we believe clients need to explore because of something they've mentioned along the way and it's something we have a passion about.

Journal Entry: *Better Never than Late*

Here is a story we heard from a friend in which the therapist's approach really created some bad feelings that were quite unnecessary:

My therapist didn't seem to want to stop. She said she had a formula, that for every month I was in therapy we needed to spend a month in the termination process. I really got a lot out of the therapy, but I didn't see the need to spend that much time saying goodbye. So I just told her that we were finished. I've come to a reasonably good spot, and I'm ready to finish. For the next few weeks, I would get brief phone calls from her saying that she was still able to meet with me. I felt like she was trying too hard to keep me as a client. And it's a shame, because even though I enjoyed the work we did, I don't think I'll go back to her when I want therapy again.

In your journal, contemplate this story in terms of the concepts we've explored in this book. What is wrong with this picture? What needs, motives, values, and acculturation strategies might the therapist be using? What possible tripping points do you see? If you were a supervisor or consultant to this therapist, what ethical principles (which Foundations) would you be addressing with her? If you were a member of an ethics committee and received a complaint about this therapist's activities, would you judge her behavior as an error in judgment or see it as an ethical violation? What is the basis for your judgment?

Client-Initiated Termination

In some therapeutic approaches, such as client-centered therapy, it is the client who generally makes the decision about termination. Ideally, the client will feel autonomous, safe, and healthy enough to suggest that therapy stop. You may think that the reaction of therapists to their clients' suggestions to stop treatment would be uniformly positive, especially when the therapy is ending with a positive outcome.

The reality, of course, is more complex. Along with feelings of happiness and fulfillment come feelings that can include sadness, rejection, resentment, and loss. Again, it is important for you to know some of your typical reactions to ending relationships. Of course, the negative feelings might be much more prominent when clients suggest ending therapy because therapy is not working for them. In essence, they want to fire us. This kind of suggestion may challenge the irrational belief, held by many therapists, that they can help anybody (Deutsch, 1984).

It's hard to stare failure in the face! It's hard to give up and refer your client to other therapists under any circumstances. But when a client suggests termination you may feel doubly bad because therapy failed, and you weren't on top of the situation enough to know exactly how bad it was! You may feel incompetent. You may feel jilted!

When referring a client to another therapist, O'Reilly (1987) suggests that therapists may experience the "transfer syndrome," which involves feelings of guilt, depression, and even relief. These feelings can be compounded by "fears of evaluation by peers or supervisors, anxiety concerning what the client might expose about him or her, and anxiety about the new placement" (Rice & Follette, 2003, p. 162). Thus, pretermination counseling sessions may be as important for therapists as they are to clients because they are opportunities for therapists to channel their anxiety into productive behaviors and to reorient their values.

When therapy fails, it is especially important for you to be aware of these emotional reactions and think about your core needs, motivations, values, virtues, and principles. How much do you value being seen as omniscient vs. being seen as facilitating client growth? Part of respecting client autonomy is respecting their judgments and choices even though they make you feel bad. These are times when your virtues of compassion and humility have to be finely tuned. If you keep the value of client welfare uppermost in your mind, you may be better able to weather the emotional storms involved in termination, especially when you get fired. Remember that handling the termination well—making excellent referrals, doing excellent pretermination counseling—can create or maintain feelings of competence even in a failed therapy. These actions thus become good integration strategies.

Too Soon

Research shows that about 20% of clients drop out of therapy prematurely (Swift & Greenberg, 2012). Dropout rates are higher for younger and less educated clients, but there are no differences in dropout rates based on theoretical orientation. However, experience does seem to make a difference; dropout rates are higher when trainees are providing the therapy.

Picture this: You are working with a client and thinking that you are just starting to make some progress. The client comes in and wants to terminate; he says that everything is fine. Here, the client may be initiating termination too soon. How do you handle this situation? How do you balance your judgment about what is in the client's best interests with their right to terminate? In other words, how do you balance the principle of beneficence with the principle of autonomy?

To deal with this situation, you need to think about some informed consent issues. For example, you need to think through how much information you provide, what options you discuss, and how much you encourage the client to continue. Sometimes this is a relatively easy matter, because you have evidence—from a competent clinical assessment—that the client's own goals have not been met. At other times, the discussion may be more of a true negotiation about goals between equal partners.

Here's a variation on the theme of the client needing more treatment: Imagine a situation in which your client's initial goals have been met and the client suggests termination. You believe, however, that the client could benefit from additional treatment. For example, the initial depression has lifted, but the client could still benefit from some assertiveness training that you are competent to provide. The decision to suggest continued therapy, when clearly the client's initial goals have been met, is a tricky one. You want to respect clients' desires, but you also want to provide information with which clients can make better decisions. The decision about how much information to provide at this point mirrors our discussion of how much information to provide at the beginning of treatment.

Food for Thought: *How to Suggest More Treatment*

You are seeing a client who has successfully dealt with the issues he came in with. However, you have strong feelings that some issues of the client's that the two of you didn't deal with in therapy are likely to cause trouble in the foreseeable future. Which of the following statements are you most likely to make? What acculturation strategies might the statement represent?

- It is my professional opinion that you need more treatment to deal with a few other issues that have arisen in the course of our work together. Because we have worked together, I would be the best person to continue to help you.
- I understand your desire to terminate. I agree that this is a great place to stop. As we do, can I share with you some impressions I have about some things that you might want to work on later, if you decide to come back or if you decide to work with somebody else?
- I'm glad we've completed our work. Good job! I wish you continued success in the future. If in the future you decide more therapy is needed, feel free to contact me.
- You really can't go yet. There are still some things you need to work on. Let's look at our calendars for next week.

Go back and consider these statements again. Might there be situations in which you are more likely to make one of the other statements? Why or Why not?

How do you know when to suggest that your client add some goals and continue therapy? Here are some possible indicators that your suggestion to continue treatment is a good one and well-done.

- The invitation to continue should not come as a surprise to your client. In fact, if the therapy has been good you might have been talking with your client all along about various directions the therapy could take.
- You should be able to offer the idea as a low-pressure suggestion, not a fiat. If you find that you really *need* the client to accept your invitation, it may be time for some consultation.

- The explanation for why the client should continue should make perfect sense— it should feel like an organic outgrowth of the work you have been doing.

Too Late

For some therapists the most difficult box in Figure 9.1 is the lower right—when therapists judge that the therapy is over (either successfully or unsuccessfully) but the client feels like therapy should go on. This may indicate client *dependency*. Clients may start talking about new goals for therapy that don't seem like they are amenable to treatment or workable for you. Or, the client may say, "You know, I think I'd like to work on my relationship with my 22nd cousin Sadie. You are the first person who really understands me." Another indication of dependency is when the client simply cannot come up with any reasons to continue but is adamant about not wanting to stop.

We have talked about ways of preventing dependency, such as being specific about goals and having a good informed consent process that includes a discussion of termination. But when it happens, the contrast between the principles of autonomy and beneficence is very stark, and the feelings and reactions we've been discussing may be especially salient. Here's one acculturation stress: Personally we may feel like we can see clients as long as they want, but from a professional standpoint, we have the obligation to terminate therapy because it is best for the client.

Green Flags: *Good Goals and Ethical Endings*

Having good goals right from the beginning makes the end of therapy easier. Consider this:

> Karyn has been working with Dr. Brooks for several months. They have been using a behavioral approach to decrease Karyn's anxiety in social situations. Karyn enjoys most of her consulting work activities, but the networking and sales was really troubling her for a long time until her therapy with Dr. Brooks.
>
> For the past several sessions, Karyn has been talking about how delighted she is with her progress, and how everything seems to be going well. She has been able to go to parties and "schmooze" quite well. Dr. Brooks says, "Well, you know Karyn, we've talked several times recently about how well you have progressed. It seems like we have accomplished your goals. In fact, our last two sessions seemed more like chatting than focused work. Maybe we ought to call the next session our last one."
>
> Karyn replies, "Oh. But I really like coming here. It just feels so comfortable to come in and just talk."

Dr. Brooks replies evenly, "It's really been a pleasure to work with you. And throughout our work, we've discussed your goals and now it seems you've met all of them. Can you think of other therapeutic goals you'd like to achieve?"

Karyn grimaces, as if she's just tasted a lemon. She knows Dr. Brooks is very straightforward, and she's finding it difficult to be confronted about ending therapy. At the same time, she knows this has been coming for a while. She recognizes that Dr. Brooks is not letting her get away with coming to therapy just because it's become a habit. "Well, when you put it that way, I guess we really are finished with our work. I just find it hard to say goodbye."

"Yes, let's consider that during our last session next week. What I hear you saying is that you agree that your goals have been met—"

"Oh, yes, definitely," Karyn says.

"But you're also saying that it's hard to leave, it's hard to say goodbye."

They spend the last few minutes of that session recapping the gains that Karyn has made. At the next session, they say their goodbyes. Dr. Brooks offers to see Karyn again when there is something to deal with. Karyn feels really good—not only that her therapist helped her with her social skills and her anxiety, but because her therapist was upfront with her about the purpose of therapy. She knows that, if problems develop in the future, there's somebody there for her.

In reality, sometimes therapists and/or clients get into a rut—it just feels good to be in psychotherapy and neither party questions the weekly appointments. However, convenience or habit is not enough to justify continued treatment. Therapists shouldn't keep seeing clients because they get used to seeing them and have nothing else to do on Tuesday afternoons. And clients should not come to therapy just because it passes the time pleasantly, or because they enjoy visiting with the therapist, or because it's a good way to avoid making friends. None of these are good reasons to continue therapy.

In sum, all these decisions have clearly to do with clinical decisions and other issues. They also have to do with your own values about what good you can provide on what level. You can provide good by doing good therapy and by allowing clients to end therapy and try out some freedom, initiative, and self-determination. You can actualize your value of doing good for clients by a prudent referral with humility and compassion.

Worst Termination Ever: Getting Complained Against

The worst-case scenario for most of us would be when clients not only inform us of their desire to terminate, but also tell us that they are filing a complaint against us with the state board or ethics committee. It is beyond the scope of this book to provide detailed suggestions for how to handle complaints against you and your practice (see Chauvin & Remley, 1996; Thomas, 2005). For now, although we hope you will never face this situation, we also want to acknowledge the possibility. It is hard to think of a more acute acculturation crisis (Berry & Kim, 1988), and this situation strikes at the heart of our values of helping and our carefully honed professional virtues. You want to be prepared for the possibility.

Some therapists may choose a separation strategy—they may discount the ethical standards they are accused of violating. Thomas wrote, "If they recognize the violation but disagree with the rule, they may believe their actions were justified and, therefore, may feel indignant and incredulous" (2005, p. 427). In our service on ethics committees, we have also seen all too often that therapists will counterattack or pathologize clients who make complaints. We have also heard about what might be extreme assimilation responses—therapists simply turn in their licenses rather than undergo an investigation of the complaint.

But there is a third response. Therapists who have been complained against still have the opportunity to take a positive approach. If we are complained against, we can take the complaint seriously and use our reasoning and choice-making skills in our response. "The ability to articulate to the board a clear understanding of mistakes and related ethical issues, and to demonstrate a commitment to rectifying problems, are likely to result in improved practices and to augment the [psychotherapist's] defense" (Thomas, 2005, p. 431).

Thomas goes on to say that the complaint process can give us an opportunity to learn. "Being the subject of a complaint may provide the impetus for initiating … changes. Time and money spent on required supervision or education may feel more worthwhile to [psychotherapists] who take an active role in determining how the experience can further their professional goals" (2005, p. 432).

At such stressful times, a positive approach includes taking time to care for ourselves—taking some time off, getting some personal support, and so forth. It also includes stepping back and perhaps re-acculturating. We may need to reexamine our core with its needs, motivations, values—what we wrote about in our ethics autobiographies and thought about when it comes to the ethical professional we want to be and how to address what seems to have gotten in the way of that goal.

Part III
The Ethical Ceiling

10

Putting It All Together
Toward Ethical Excellence

"How do you get to Carnegie Hall? Practice, practice, practice."
Old joke, attributed to Henny Youngman

Here we are at the end of the book—you've finished the tour of the mansion (the profession and your developing professional/ethical identity). You've walked up the spiral staircase of making ethical decisions. Sometimes you hung on to the handrails when they were there and other times you reached for them only to realize— Nope!—they're absent. Ethical guides and codes don't (can't) address every issue. While climbing the staircase you've noticed that some steps aren't level—in fact, they're downright slippery. Tripping and falling are easy outcomes. After all, psychotherapists, like all humans, can make ethical mistakes because of faulty thinking, emotional involvements, conflicts of interest, and other factors.

Some of the rooms represent your core, which includes your needs, motivations, and values. Other rooms represent the profession, with its values, traditions, processes, knowledge, and ethics. There was a third set of rooms where you began to bring furniture from the personal rooms and professional rooms to see what the combination feels and looks like. At times you may have felt comfortable in the mansion: "This is home and it feels good." At other times you may have felt uncomfortable, anxious, maybe even frustrated: "This doesn't feel like home and I'm not sure it ever will." Be patient: Your professional/ethical identity will continue to form and your acculturation to the profession is a life-long process.

As we stated in the Introduction, we wanted to help you come to know what is important to you and what is important about ethics and ethical identity. We also wanted to help you understand ethical thinking, choice making, pitfalls (tripping points), and behaviors. In this chapter, we provide an opportunity to review what you have learned about yourself, your ethical identity, ethical thinking and choice making, and your acculturation to the profession.

You and Your Professional/Ethical Identity

Exploring your core has likely revealed some needs, motivations, and values that were hidden or unknown. What was that exploration like? What activities did you (a) enjoy—and why—and what activities did you (b) find challenging—and why?

We encourage you to do some writing to tap into what you now know about you and your core.

Journal Entry: *Your Current View of You as an Ethical Person*

In the Introduction we shared our definition of ethical identity: your view of self as an ethical person. In Chapter 1, we asked you to reflect on who you are, what it means to be you, and about your needs, motivations, values, and virtues. Look back at what you wrote. What would you tweak, add, or subtract? What is your current view of self as an ethical person? Choose one of the following ways to express your current view:

- Write a short (no more than 250 words) addendum to your description of your ethical self—who you are at your core—the foundation of your professional/ethical identity.
- Write a letter to yourself. You might share your observations and thoughts about your growth as an ethical person and professional. You might share your wishes and hopes for the next steps in your ethical growth. You might craft a plan of action to accomplish these steps.
- Construct a visual representation of your ethical self—a drawing, a painting, a sculpture, or a word cloud—from something that you have composed thus far in your exploration of who you are at the core.

On the professional side, you've explored the ethical landscape of psychotherapy, including some cultural aspects of the profession: social responsibility, confidentiality, competence, informed consent, boundaries, self-care, supervision, and foundational principles. You've considered green flags, red flags, and tripping points. You've paused to think: What do I think about that? What do I need to do about that? What do I want to do about that? What sources of guidance are there?

Think back to the two examples Sharon shared in the Introduction about the interactive nature of our core and professional culture and how that manifested in two students. One student decided to leave the program because of a clash of values between her core and the profession. The other student had a clash with his family culture and decided to strengthen his values, motivations, and choices around keeping things private or confidential. Both students made the right choice. You may have had some experiences where you realized, "Wow, that (whatever it is) doesn't work for me anymore. I'm more aware, I've grown, I've changed." You've discovered, uncovered, or embraced parts of your core identity which influence how you see and understand the profession and its culture. In turn the profession's ethics and culture have influenced you at your core.

You and Your Ethical Acculturation to the Profession

In Chapter 3, we introduced the idea of ethical acculturation and explored how we adapt to our new professional culture. This adaptation occurs along two dimensions: (a) maintenance and (b) contact and participation. The maintenance dimension includes, "What will I keep from my personal ethical/moral identity (my core) as I enter this new profession?" The contact and participation dimension includes, "What in the professional culture do I see having value and therefore want to identify with and adopt?" These two dimensions or tasks happen simultaneously. Taking time to reflect on your core makes the maintenance task clearer. Coming to know and evaluate the professional culture and deciding what you want to embrace or adopt addresses the second task, contact and participation.

Food for Thought: *I Don't See or Think About Things the Way I Used to*

Think about some discussions, situations, and/or observations where you noticed yourself thinking, "That concerns me now," or "Now I see that is ethically problematic. I need to think more carefully about what I might or should do." What has prompted these changes? Was it your personal self influencing your professional/ ethical identity, or vice versa? How has the process strengthened your ethical/ professional identity?

As you continue to develop your professional ethical identity, we encourage you to pause and think about which acculturation strategy you are choosing. If it is not integration, but one of the other three strategies, ask yourself why. "Why am I choosing this strategy? What needs to change for me to move toward integration? Do I need to realign or express my personal motivations and values to honor my professional obligations better? Am I burned out? Am I trying to meet my personal needs through my clients and their success?" Keep these keys in mind:

- Becoming ethically excellent is a life-long journey.
- Professional obligations and personal demands sometimes compete—that's a reality.
- Set the integration strategy as your goal, and then be patient with yourself.
- Remember that perfection is an illusion.
- Let your humility take over, and seek out ethical support and challenge.
- Consultation is one of your best professional steps. Make it a frequent and usual part of your professional life.

Railings, Tripping Points, and Making Ethical Choices

Our mansion includes many railings (ethical codes and ethical foundations) to guide and support us as we traverse stairs. But as we've seen, railings may not exist, they may change, or the stairs may be slippery. In Chapter 4, we explored the foundational principles that all psychotherapy disciplines endorse about the psychotherapy relationship, including issues of competence. We also noted these truths:

- The psychotherapy relationship is complex and fragile.
- Clients have the right to expect that we have the skill and expertise to help them—that they will be better off having worked with us.

We are more likely to act ethically and effectively if we can anticipate, prevent, and mitigate the effects of tripping points. As you look back and reflect on the tripping points, think about three categories of responses: (a) "Not me. I don't really see this being a problem." (b) "This one has my name written all over it." (c) "This could be a problem. I'll have to be aware." Then, remember the bias blind spot, which will allow you to assume that there are NO tripping points in category a! And: situational stresses may move lots of tripping points from category c to category b.

We hope it has been useful for you to consider tripping points and acculturation strategies as you develop your choice-making skills. In Chapter 4, we presented a way to consider choices based on Rest's four components of ethical behavior. In the cases below, see how you might use these four components as you choose the ethical course(s) of action. To refresh your memory, here are the four components and some of the questions.

Component 1—Ethical Sensitivity

- What strikes you as needing some type of response or makes you uncomfortable?
- What is that gut response about?
- What makes you think, "Uh-oh, this doesn't seem right"? or "Yes, this seems good or right"?

- What are the issues related to diversity and equity? To differences in identities between my client and me? To oppression or discrimination?
- How do your points of privilege affect your ethical sensitivity to this issue?
- What are the possible choices to pursue?
- Who will be affected by the different choices?

Component 2—Formulating an Ethical Plan

- What do you know about the situation? What else do you need to know?
  - What are the facts of the case?
  - What are the contextual issues?
- What do ethics codes and other guides have to say about this situation? What ethical standards conflict in this situation?
- What are the legal issues involved?
- With whom should you consult? Who would help you see multiple perspectives?
- What do you need to explain or share with the client about the ethical issue?
- If you were the client, what would you hope the psychotherapist would do?

Component 3—Ethical Motivation and Competing Values

- What are your personal needs and motivations in this situation?
- What are your professional values and obligations in this situation?
- To what extent is there an overlap and match between the two, and to what extent is there a conflict?
- Are there personal and/or professional values that need to be reorganized or reprioritized? If yes, what are they and how do they need to be addressed?
- With whom might you consult to see the conflicts as clearly as possible?

Component 4—Ethical Follow-Through

- To whom and/or what (e.g., ethics code, law) must you be accountable? To whom do you want to be accountable?
- Who in your professional circles can encourage or support you to do the right thing?
- What personal and professional values do you need to draw upon to implement the choice?
- What are the possible deterrents for you in following through on what you need to do?
- As you implement this choice, what do you need to let the client know?

Cases for Exploration

Here are a few cases for you to practice your choice-making process. After the cases we encourage you to do some more reflecting.

The Case of the Indispensable Insurance

You are seeing a client for some marital problems. He's a little sad, a little anxious, but doesn't really come close to fitting any psychiatric diagnosis. He does not have enough money to be able to afford therapy without insurance, and his insurance will not pay for therapy without a diagnosis. You are pretty sure your therapeutic approach will be successful. At the same time, your own budget is tight and you really can't afford to have someone who can't pay taking up one of your billable hours.

Here's a variation of the story: You are doing marital therapy for the client and his wife, but the insurance only covers individual therapy.

Here are some questions to get you started: How would you report your work to the insurance company? What if the client was one symptom shy of a reimbursable diagnosis? Would it be ethical or not to report that you were doing "individual therapy" for the husband with the wife as a "collateral contact"?

What tripping points and situational pressures might be operative for you? What if you were working at an agency and your supervisor asked/demanded that you complete the diagnosis? Might you be thinking something like this?: "Giving a diagnosis is just a formality. This is really what insurance is for. Anyway, my treatment will save the insurance company money in the long run by preventing my client from having a full-blown depression."

Continue with the choice-making model. Bear in mind that intentionally assigning a diagnosis that is not accurate is unethical—it is insurance fraud. Such a behavior might be evidence of a separation or marginalization strategy.

The Case of the Relative Referral

You are a very well-trained and competent family therapist in a small city. You have been seeing a couple, off and on, over a period of 5 years. They came to you when their marriage hit a rough spot. Your typical approach is solution-focused and thus far you have had good success. Based on your ongoing assessment, the relationship seems to be getting stronger.

One day the husband calls you and asks for a referral for himself. He would like to go into individual therapy with somebody who uses the same approach you do. He says, "I'd come to see you because I really like how you work, but I know that I can't because I'm already seeing you as part of a couple."

"That's right," you answer, sure of your ethical ground. "That would be a conflict of interest for me and a multiple relationship for us. But I'll think about some possible referrals and give you a couple names of people I trust."

The next day you call the client with names of the best two therapists in town who use the same approach you do. "The first person is Samuel Howard, an excellent therapist."

"I know him!" your client says. "He's a tennis buddy of mine!"

"Well, that leaves him out, obviously." You share your other name—someone your client is not familiar with. You're just about to end the call on that successful note when your client says, "I'd really like one or two more names, just in case I don't get along with this person. I'd feel much more comfortable with a choice of folks."

"Let me think about it and get back to you." You already know that there are very few people in town who use your approach. The good news is that there is one more person you know who is a good therapist—well trained, seasoned, very ethical, and able to be very successful with your client. The bad news is: this person is your spouse/partner!

Here are some of your alternative courses of action:

- You could tell your client you don't have any other referrals to offer.
- You could give the client your spouse's name as a referral and not tell the client you are related to the person (you have different last names). After all, you and your spouse never talk about the details of cases you are seeing, including identities, so there is little if any danger of either of you finding out things you shouldn't know.
- You could give the client the referral and explain to him that the therapist is your spouse. You could explain your policy as a professional couple about not sharing names or details about clients, and offer to answer any questions the client has.
- You could discuss with your client the possibility of working with someone who has a different approach and that this would probably yield a larger list of referrals.

What other options might there be? What are the pros and cons for each option? Which options would represent—for you—integration, assimilation, and separation strategies? Why? Which one appears to be the *most* ethical course of action? Which option appears to be the *least* ethical?

What if the referral was for a family member whom you were not seeing—a father, mother, sibling, son, or daughter? How would that change the issues and considerations? What other facts of the case would alter the choices you make?

The Case of the Tele-Transition

One of your supervisees contacts you and shares the following situation: "I have this client and we've done some really good work. The client told me, 'I really appreciate our work together. I know I am in a better space'." Your supervisee continues: "A few minutes later the client says to me, 'I know we've talked a little bit about my relationship with my boss. I really want to be successful but it seems like I can't make a good connection with them. Could we work on this? I really appreciate the way we've connected'."

You and your supervisee believe the client's goal is reasonable and your supervisee's therapeutic modality will work well. You give the green light for the work to continue. The second week into working on the new goal, life takes its own course. A pandemic has occurred, and your supervisee and their client cannot meet face to face. Your supervisee contacts you and asks for some guidance. The client wants to continue to work and suggests they meet via Zoom. Your supervisee has read about telehealth—so have you—but not tried it. In fact, you are scheduled to attend a telehealth workshop in the future. What choices do you have, and what do you conclude?

Reflections on the Cases

When you think about these cases (and any others), think about this: In which cases did your personal and professional needs, motivations, and values seem to overlap the most? You may have found it easier to identify what seemed ethically right and to see good integration strategies.

You know what we're going to ask next: What cases prompted more conflict between your personal and professional values, needs, and motivations? What were the conflicts? Did you think, "The profession is making too big of a deal out of this issue"? Or maybe, "Why doesn't the code talk about this? It seems really important to client wellbeing."

Did you experience acculturation stress with any of the cases? If yes, which acculturation strategy did you lean toward implementing and why?

Before we head to our last sections, we want to remind you of the following points. First, sometimes what we need to do is not all that clear. Second, ethical decision making takes effort. Third, sometimes a clear choice is not the best—it may represent a tripping point. Fourth, the profession of psychotherapy is complex. Fifth, making and implementing ethical choices doesn't always feel good. In fact, many times our emotions may be mixed.

Journal Entry: *Cultures*

Go back to the journal entry you completed in Chapter 4: "My Current Location on the Road to Multicultural Competence." Notice the three cultures you feel you know a lot about and the three you know little or nothing about. Now, go back through this chapter, and the rest of the book, and find several exercises that didn't have any specific reference to culture. Make the people in those exercises members of each of the cultures you know a lot about. How does that change things? Do this exercise again and make the people in the exercises a member of the cultures you know little or nothing about. What changes? What steps might you take to improve your multicultural competence?

Ethics Autobiography—Update

As your final task for this book, it's time to revise your ethics autobiography. Re-read your autobiography with an eye toward a revision that will serve you for the next phase of your training or career. What parts of the autobiography do you need to change? How might you work toward increasing your use of integration strategies? Where do you need work on virtues, values, and social awareness? In addition, what behaviors do you give up or alter by being a professional (e.g., dating, sex, gossip, self-disclosure)? What do you gain by being a professional (e.g., watching people grow, appropriate use of knowledge and skill, gratitude, money)?

Add one more section to the autobiography: Make a list of your strengths, those aspects of ethical acculturation in which you find yourself articulate and confident. Then, make a list of the other aspects—those for which the words, feelings, and thoughts do not come so quickly. There is your list of what you can do to facilitate your development as a professional.

Toward Ethical Excellence

Here are a couple final points we want to share with you before you close the book. First, this book is ending, but your professional journey of continuing to develop your professional/ethical identity is not. Second, your experience of exploring the mansion, climbing the staircase, and visiting different rooms was meant to help you build a foundation for your ethical identity. There is no endpoint because we continue to change, to gain insight, and to improve our virtues, behaviors, and acculturation strategies. Striving for excellence is a process that keeps us going as professionals. Third, we encourage you to look back at this book, your responses to the activities, and your ethics autobiography on a regular basis to reflect on your growth and new challenges.

A Final Word

The relationship between authors and readers is yet another type of professional relationship with its own set of expectations, role obligations, and boundaries. We hope we have fulfilled our obligation to provide you with an experience that has enhanced your development and allowed you to fulfill your own obligations—to yourself and to the profession. We hope that the time we have spent together exploring what is in your core, the profession, tripping points, and the ethical foundations will have long-term benefits for you and your clients. We wish you much success and our last invitation to you is to share your reactions to and experiences with this book with us. Here are our email addresses:

Sharon: sharon.anderson@colostate.edu
Mitch: mitchell.handelsman@ucdenver.edu

Appendix A

Possible Information to Be Shared with Clients

Much of this information is from Pomerantz & Handelsman, 2004.

Issues to Address About the Logistics of Therapy

- How often you'll meet for therapy
- The length and time of each session
- How appointment times are scheduled (phone, email, texts, etc.)
- Your usual availability during the week
- How appointments can be changed when necessary
- How to reach you in case of an emergency
- Your back-up coverage when you aren't available
- Whether or not you are able and willing to do therapy over the phone or the internet
- Your fee structure and how you handle no-shows
- How you are set up to receive payments
- How you will handle the situation if the client falls behind in payments
- Your policy for raising fees
- If the client decides to use insurance:
    - how much and what kind of information you will be required to share with the insurance company (diagnosis, symptoms, other information)
    - the impact the insurance company can have on the therapy
    - the possible issues if the insurance company and you disagree about treatment

Issues to Address About the Therapeutic Process

- The therapeutic approach you propose based on the client's goals and concerns
- What the research says about your approach and the client's concern
- Your therapeutic approach and how you understand change
- Your understanding of how issues of discrimination, injustice, and systematic oppression impact mental health

- How your therapeutic approach is structured and whether or not you follow preplanned format
- Any estimate you have about the length of therapy
- How the two of you will:
  1. measure therapeutic progress
  2. know when your work together is done
  3. know when therapy is not working and the options available for the client
- The benefits of your therapeutic approach
- The risks of your therapeutic approach
- Assessments or tests you might have the client complete
- The types of issues or concerns that you don't feel competent to address
- Your connection(s) with prescribing physicians
- The percentage of your clients that improve and how you know this information
- The percentage of your clients that don't improve and even get worse and how you know this information
- The other types of therapy that work (according to research) with their concerns or goals
- The risks and benefits of NO therapy for people with their type of concern or goal

Issues to Address About Ethics Policies

- Professional organizations you belong to
- The codes of ethics you use or you are bound to (be ready to hand a copy of your current ethics code to your client in case he or she asks for a copy)
- Ethical guidelines you use regarding confidentiality
- The kinds of records you keep and who has access to them (insurance companies, supervisors, employers, others)
- The conditions where you are required to breach confidentiality
- How you will handle confidentiality when it comes to family members
- How HIPAA and other governmental regulations influence confidentiality of your records
- How you handle boundary issues or multiple relationships with clients
- Who the client can talk with if they have a complaint about therapy which can't be worked out between the two of you

Issues About You and Self-Disclosure

- Your policy about therapist self-disclosure
- The kind(s) of degree(s) you have and what they were in
- The institution(s) you received them from

- Your license as a psychotherapist
- The number of years you have been doing psychotherapy
- How long you have been helping people with the client's sort of problem(s)
- The entity that regulates your psychotherapy practice
- Other credentials you have acquired that suggest more training or expertise
- If you are under supervision, who your supervisor is and how the client can contact him or her
- What are some of your basic values that guide your work and your life?
- Do you work from a religious/spiritual framework? If so, how does that show up in your practice? What will it look like in session?

Appendix B

Policy Areas

These are some of the areas in which you might want to have written policies. Some of these will be familiar, as we've talked about them in this book. Others will be new to you. As you formulate each policy, be sure to consider all the work you've done exploring (a) your core, (b) your acculturation tasks, stresses, and strategies, (c) the guides you have for your choices, including values, virtues, and codes, and (d) your potential tripping points. You will need to adapt your general policies depending on:

- The context of your practice (agency, group private practice, etc.)
- The range of your clients (diagnosis, SES, gender, religion, ethnic group, etc.)
- The types of clients and client issues you consider difficult

Remember that this is not an exhaustive list of policy areas (although it is exhausting…). But it will get you started, no?

1. How do I dress?
2. What objects (pictures, diplomas, awards, political material, etc.) do I display in my office?
3. How do I determine my competence to treat a client?
4. Clients whom I am incompetent to treat
5. Forms of address—what do I want to be called by clients?
6. Pre-appointment information to send to clients, receive from them
7. Use of different technologies to contact and serve clients
8. Informed consent
   a. What do I tell all clients?
   b. What are the risks of my therapy?
   c. How do I tell clients the information they need to know?
   d. How do I address client questions?
   e. How do I assess what information particular clients might need to know?
   f. How do I document consent? Refusal? Assent?
   g. Contracts
9. What rights do clients have?
   a. Consent
   b. Termination
   c. Second opinion

    d. Asking questions

    e. Rights to records

10. How do I formulate the goals of treatment?

11. Coverage for vacations, weekends, other absences

12. Emergencies

13. Extra-therapy contacts

    a. Phone calls

    b. Texts

    c. Emails

    d. Social media

    e. Collateral contacts

14. Invitations from clients for extra-therapy contact (social events, life events)

    a. What are my criteria for accepting and rejecting invitations?

15. Confidentiality

    a. Storing client information

    b. Releases of information

    c. Privilege and other legal issues

    d. Requests for information from others

    e. How do I send records?

    f. What is my complete list of exceptions to confidentiality, including abuse reporting, court orders, and other legal requirements?

16. Records

    a. Storage—computer, files, etc.

    b. Disposal

    c. Retention of records

    d. Deleting obsolete records

    e. Sharing records with clients, colleagues

    f. Plans for moving, retiring, death

    g. What is the format of my records?

    h. What are the components of my records?

17. Accepting and giving gifts

18. Finances

    a. Fees for sessions, other contacts, emergencies, phone calls, testimony, etc.

    b. Raising fees

    c. Negotiating fees for new clients, clients' whose circumstances change, etc.

    d. Missed and cancelled appointments

    e. Billing and collecting fees

    f. Bartering

19. Advertising and public statements

20. Safety issues

    a. How do I deal with clients who seem to be getting angry?

    b. How do I deal with suicidal gestures, threats, behaviors?

    c. How do I deal with threats from clients, others?

21. Termination and referral
    a. How do I inform clients about the conditions under which termination and/or referral takes place?
    b. How do I terminate?
    c. How do I refer?
    d. How do I conduct pretermination (pre-referral) counseling?
22. Knowledge of unprofessional conduct by colleagues
    a. How do I talk with colleagues about concerns I have about their behavior?
    b. What is my threshold for reporting the unethical conduct of colleagues?
23. If I am sued or complained against to an ethics committee
    a. Who am I going to call?
        i. Attorney
        ii. Insurance carrier
        iii. Risk management office at your agency
        iv. Therapist
        v. Family
        vi. Colleagues
24. Touching
    a. What do I consider to be beneficial and not harmful?
    b. How will I know if my initial consideration is in error?

References

Abeles, N. (1980). Teaching ethical principles by means of values confrontations. *Psychotherapy: Theory, Research and Practice*, 17(4), 384–391.

Ahia, C. E., & Martin, D. (1993). The danger-to-self-or-others exception to confidentiality. In T. P. Remley (Ed.), *ACA legal series* (Vol. 9). Alexandria, VA: American Counseling Association.

American Association for Marriage and Family Therapy. (2015). *Code of ethics*. https://www.aamft.org/Legal_Ethics/Code_of_Ethics.aspx

American Counseling Association. (2014). *ACA code of ethics*. Alexandria, VA: Author.

American Psychological Association. (2017). *Ethical principles of psychologists and code of conduct*. https://www.apa.org/ethics/code

Anderson, S. K. (2015). Morally sensitive professionals. In D. S. Mower, P. Vandenberg, & W. L. Robison (Eds.), *Developing moral sensitivity* (pp. 188–204). New York: Routledge.

Anderson, S. K. (2018). An awakening to privilege, oppression, and discrimination: Sharon's story. In S. K. Anderson & V. A. Middleton (Eds.), *Explorations in diversity: Examining the complexities of privilege, discrimination, and oppression* (pp. 3–8). Oxford University Press.

Anderson, S. K., & Kitchener, K. S. (1996). A critical incident study of nonromantic/nonsexual relationships between psychologists and former clients. *Professional Psychology: Research and Practice*, 27(1), 59–66.

Anderson, S. K., & Kitchener, K. S. (1998). Nonsexual post-therapy relationships: a conceptual framework to assess ethical risks. *Professional Psychology: Research and Practice*, 29(1), 91–99.

Anderson, S. K., Wagoner, H., & Moore, G. K. (2006). Ethical choice: An outcome of being, blending, and doing. In P. Williams & S. K. Anderson (Eds.), *Law and ethics in coaching: How to solve and avoid difficult problems in your practice* (pp. 39–61). Hoboken, NJ: John Wiley & Sons.

Appelbaum, P., & Gutheil, T. (2019). *Clinical handbook of psychiatry and the law* (5th ed.). Philadelphia, PA: Lippincott, Williams & Wilkins.

Asay, P. A., & Lal, A. (2014). Who's googled whom? Trainees' internet and online social networking experiences, behaviors, and attitudes with clients and supervisors. *Training and Education in Professional Psychology*, 8(2), 105–111. doi:10.1037/tep0000035

Ashby, G. A., O'Brien, A., Bowman, D., Hooper, C., Stevens, T., & Lousada, E. (2015). Should psychiatrists "google" their patients? *BJPsych Bulletin*, 39(6), 278–283. doi:10.1192/pb.bp.114.047555

Auxier, C. R., Hughes, F. R., & Kline, W. B. (2003). Identity development in counselors-in-training. *Counselor Education & Supervision*, 43(1), 25–38.

Baird, B. N. (1999). *The internship, practicum, and filed placement handbook*. Upper Saddle River, NJ: Prentice Hall.

Barnett, J. E. (2007). Whose boundaries are they anyway? *Professional Psychology: Research and Practice*, 38(4), 401–405.

Barnett, J. E. (2015). A practical ethics approach to boundaries and multiple relationships in psychotherapy. *British Psychological Society Psychotherapy Section Review*, 56(1), 27–37.

Barnett, J. E., & Molson, C. H. (2014). Clinical supervision of psychotherapy: Essential ethics issues for supervisors and supervisees. *Journal of Clinical Psychology: In Session*, 70(11), 1051–1061.

Barnett, J. E., Wise, E. H., Johnson-Greene, D., & Bucky, S. F. (2007). Informed consent: Too much of a good thing or not enough? *Professional Psychology: Research and Practice*, 38(2), 179–186.

Bashe, A., Anderson, S. K., Handelsman, M. M., & Klevansky, R. (2007). An acculturation model for ethics training: The ethics autobiography and beyond. *Professional Psychology: Research and Practice*, 38(1), 60–67.

Batson, C. D., Kobrynowicz, J. L., Dinnerstain, H., Kampf, C., & Wilson, A. D. (1997). In a very different voice: Unmasking moral hypocrisy. *Journal of Personality and Social Psychology*, 72(6), 1335–1348.

Bazerman, M. H., & Tenbrunsel, A. E. (2011). *Blind spots: Why we fail to do what's right and what to do about it*. Princeton, NJ: Princeton University Press.

Bazerman, M. H., Tenbrunsel, A. E., & Wade-Benzoni, K. (1998). Negotiating with yourself and losing: Making decisions with competing internal preferences. *Academy of Management Review*, 23(2), 225–241.

Beahrs, J., & Gutheil, T. (2001). Informed consent in psychotherapy. *American Journal of Psychiatry*, 158(4–10). doi:10.1176/appi.ajp.158.1.4

Beddoe, L. (2017). Harmful supervision: A commentary. *The Clinical Supervisor*, 36(1), 88–101.

Bergus, G. R., Chapman, G. B., Levy, B. T., Ely, J. W., & Oppliger, R. A. (1998). Clinical diagnosis and the order of information. *Medical Decision Making*, 18(4), 412–417.

Bernard, J. L., & Jara, C. S. (1986). The failure of clinical psychology graduate students to apply understood ethical principles. *Professional Psychology: Research and Practice*, 17(4), 313–315.

Bernard, J. L., Murphy, M., & Little, M. (1987). The failure of clinical psychologists to apply understood ethical principles. *Professional Psychology: Research and Practice*, 18(5), 489–491.

Bernard, J. M., & Goodyear, R. K. (2014). *The fundamentals of clinical supervision* (5th ed.). New York: Pearson.

Bernard, J. M., & Goodyear, R. K. (2019). *Fundamentals of clinical supervision* (6th ed.). New York: Pearson.

Berry, J. W. (1980). Acculturation as varieties of adaptation. In A. M. Padilla (Ed.), *Acculturation: Theory, models, and some new findings* (pp. 9–25). Boulder, CO: Westview Press.

Berry, J. W. (2003). Conceptual approaches to acculturation. In K. M. Chun, P. B. Organista, & G. Marin (Eds.), *Acculturation: Advances in theory, measurement, and applied research* (pp. 17–37). Washington, DC: American Psychological Association.

Berry, J. W., & Kim, U. (1988). Acculturation and mental health. In P. R. Dasen, J. W. Berry, & N. Sartorius (Eds.), *Health and cross-cultural psychology* (pp. 207–236). Newbury Park, NY: Sage.

Berry, J. W., & Sam, D. L. (1997). Acculturation and adaptation. In J. W. Berry, M. H. Segall, & C. Kagitçibasi (Eds.), *Handbook of cross-cultural psychology* (pp. 291–326). Needham Heights, MA: Allyn and Bacon.

Betan, E. J., & Stanton, A. L. (1999). Fostering ethical willingness: Integrating emotional and contextual awareness with rational analysis. *Professional Psychology: Research and Practice*, 30(3), 295–301.

Birch, J. (1990). The context-setting function of the video "consent" form. *Journal of Family Therapy*, 12(3), 281–286.

Birchmore, T. (2015). Letter from the editor. *British Psychological Society Psychotherapy Section Review*, 56(1), 1–2.

Blasi, A. (1984). Moral identity: Its role in moral functioning. In W. M. Kurtines & J. J. Gewirtz (Eds.), *Morality, moral behavior and moral development* (pp. 128–139). New York: John Wiley & Sons.

Blumenfeld, W. J., & Raymond, D. (2000). Prejudice and discrimination. In M. Adams, W. J. Blumenfeld, R. Castaneda, H. W. Hackman, M. L. Peters, & X. Zuniga (Eds.), *Readings for diversity and social justice* (pp. 35–49). New York: Routledge.

Bok, S. (1989). *Secrets: On the ethics of concealment and revelation.* New York: Vintage Books.

Borders, L. D., Glosoff, H. L., Welfare, L. E., Hays, D. G., DeKruyf, L., Fernando, D. M., & Page, B. (2014). Best practices in clinical supervision: Evolution of a counseling specialty. *The Clinical Supervisor*, 33(1), 26–44.

Braaten, E. B., & Handelsman, M. M. (1997). Client preferences for informed consent information. *Ethics & Behavior*, 7(4), 311–328.

Braaten, E. B., Otto, S., & Handelsman, M. M. (1993). What do people want to know about psychotherapy? *Psychotherapy*, 30(4), 565–570.

Branstetter, S. A., & Handelsman, M. M. (2000). Graduate teaching assistants: Ethical training, beliefs, and practices. *Ethics & Behavior*, 10(1), 27–50.

Brown, L. S. (1994). Boundaries in feminist therapy: A conceptual formulation. *Women & Therapy*, 15(1), 29–38.

Bucher, R., & Stelling, J. G. (1977). *Becoming professional.* Beverly Hills, CA: Sage.

Buckley, P., Karasu, T. B., & Charles, E. (1981). Psychotherapists view their personal therapy. *Psychotherapy: Theory, Research, and Practice*, 18(3), 299–305.

Burke, P. J. (2003). Introduction. In P. J. Burke, T. J. Owens, R. T. Serpe, & P. A. Thoits (Eds.), *Advances in identity theory and research* (pp. 1–10). New York: Kluwer Academic/Plenum.

Canadian Psychological Association. (2017). *Canadian code of ethics for psychologists* (4th ed.). Ottawa, ON: Author.

Carifio, M. S., & Hess, A. K. (1987). Who is the ideal supervisor? *Professional Psychology: Research and Practice*, 18(3), 244–250.

Chauvin, J. C., & Remley, T. P., Jr. (1996). Responding to allegations of unethical conduct. *Journal of Counseling & Development*, 74(6), 563–568.

Clark, C. R. (1993). Social responsibility ethics: Doing right, doing good, doing well. *Ethics and Behavior*, 3(3–4), 303–328.

Corey, C., Corey, M. S., & Callanan, P. (2007). *Issues and ethics in the helping professions* (7th ed.). Belmont, CA: Brooks Cole.

Cornish, J., Kitchener, K. S., & Barnett, J. (2008, August). Supervisor and Supervisee ethical expectations –What goes on behind closed doors? Paper presentation at the 116th Annual Convention of the American Psychological Association, Boston, MA.

Cottone, R. R. (2012). Ethical decision making in mental health contexts: Representative models and an organizational framework. In S. J. Knapp, M. C. Gottlieb, M. M. Handelsman, & L. D. VandeCreek (Eds.), *APA handbook of ethics in psychology, Vol. 1. Moral foundations and common themes* (pp. 99–121). American Psychological Association. doi:10.1037/13271-004

Cottone, R. R., Tarvydas, V., & Claus, R. E. (2007). Ethical decision-making process. In R. R. Cottone & V. M. Tarvydas (Eds.), *Counseling ethics and decision making* (3rd ed.). Upper Saddle River, NJ: Pearson Merrill Prentice Hall.

Cottone, R. R., & Tarvydas, V. M. (Eds.) (2007). *Counseling ethics and decision making* (3rd ed.). Upper Saddle River, NJ: Pearson Merrill Prentice Hall.

Cottone, R. R., & Tarvydas, V. M. (2016). *Ethics and decision making in counseling and psychotherapy* (4th ed.). New York: Springer.

Coyne, J. C., & Widiger, T. A. (1978). Toward a participatory model of psychotherapy. *Professional Psychology*, 9(4), 700–701.

Crawford, M. J., Thana, L., Farquharson, L., Palmer, L., Hancock, E., Bassett, P., ... Parry, G. D. (2016). Patient experience of negative effects of psychological treatment: Results of a national survey. *The British Journal of Psychiatry*, 208(3), 60–265. doi:10.1192/bjp. bp.114.162628

Cruess, S. R., Johnston, S., & Cruess, R. L. (2004). "Profession": A working definition for medical educators. *Teaching and Learning in Medicine*, 16(1), 74–76.

Davis, D. (2008). *Terminating therapy: A professional guide to ending on a positive note*. Hoboken, NJ: Wiley.

Davis, D. D., & Younggren, J. N. (2009). Ethical competence in psychotherapy termination. *Professional Psychology: Research and Practice*, 40(6), 572–578.

De Golia, S. G., & Corcoran, K. M. (Eds.). (2019). *Supervision in psychiatric practice: Practical approaches across venues and providers*. Washington, DC: American Psychiatric Pub.

Deutsch, C. J. (1984). Self-reported sources of stress among psychotherapists. *Professional Psychology: Research and Practice*, 15(6), 835–845.

DiLillo, D., & Gale, E. B. (2011). To google or not to google: Graduate students' use of the internet to access personal information about clients. *Training and Education in Professional Psychology*, 5(3), 160–166. doi:10.1037/a0024441

Driscoll, J. M. (1992). Keeping covenants and confidences sacred: One point of view. *Journal of Counseling and Development*, 70(6), 704–708.

Dsubanko-Obermayr, K., & Baumann, U. (2010). Informed consent in psychotherapy: Demands and reality. *Psychotherapy Research*, 8(3), 231–247.

Dunn, R., Callahan, J. L., Farnsworth, J. K., & Watkins, C. E., Jr. (2017). A proposed framework for addressing supervisee–supervisor value conflict. *The Clinical Supervisor*, 36(2), 203–222.

Dunning, D. (2011). The Dunning–Kruger effect: On being ignorant of one's own ignorance. *Advances in Experimental Social Psychology*, 44, 247–296. doi:10.1016/B978-0-12-385522-0.00005-6

Eichenberg, C., & Herzberg, P. Y. (2016). Do therapists google their patients? A survey among psychotherapists. *Journal of Medical Internet Research*, 18(1), e3. doi:l0.2l96/jmir.4306

Ellis, M. (2017). Narratives of harmful clinical supervision. *The Clinical Supervisor*, 36(1), 20–87.

Ellis, M. V. (1991). Critical incidents in clinical supervision and in supervisor supervision: Assessing supervisory issues. *Journal of Counseling Psychology*, 38(3), 342–349.

Epley, N., & Dunning, D. (2000). Feeling "holier than thou": Are self-serving assessments produced by errors in self- or social perception? *Journal of Personality and Social Psychology*, 79(6), 861–875.

Fisher, C. B., & Oransky, M. (2008). Informed consent to psychotherapy: Protecting the dignity and respecting the autonomy of patients. *Journal of Clinical Psychology*, 64(5), 576–588. doi:10.1002/jclp.20472

Friedlander, M. L. (2015). Use of relational strategies to repair alliance ruptures: How responsive supervisors train responsive psychotherapists. *Psychotherapy*, 52(2), 174.

Furman, R. (2005). White male privilege in the context of my life. In S. K. Anderson & V. A. Middleton (Eds.), *Explorations in privilege, oppression and discrimination* (pp. 25–29). Belmont, CA: Thomson Brooks/Cole.

Gabbard, G. O. (1989). *Sexual exploitation in professional relationships*. Washington, DC: American Psychiatric Association.

Gabbard, G. O., & Lester, E. P. (2003). *Boundaries and boundary violations in psychoanalysis*. Washington, DC: American Psychiatric Publishing.

Gilley, J. W., Anderson, S. K., & Gilley, A. (2008). Ethics in human resources. In S. Quatro (Ed.), *Executive ethics: Ethical dilemmas and challenges for the C-suite*. Charlotte, NC: Information Age Publishing.

Gladwell, M. (2000). *The tipping point: How little things can make a big difference*. New York: Little, Brown, and Company.

Glaser, R. D., & Thorpe, J. S. (1986). Unethical intimacy: A survey of sexual contact and advances between psychology educators and female graduate students. *American Psychologist*, 41(1), 43–51.

Gottlieb, M. C., Handelsman, M. M., & Knapp, S. (2013). A model for integrated ethics consultation. *Professional Psychology: Research and Practice*, 44(5), 307–313.

Grater, H. A. (1985). Stages in psychotherapy supervision: From therapy skills to skilled therapist. *Professional Psychology: Research and Practice*, 16(5), 605–610.

Grove, A. S. (2002). *Swimming across: A memoir*. New York: Grand Central.

Gutheil, T. G., & Gabbard, G. O. (1993). The concept of boundaries in clinical practice: Theoretical and risk-management dimensions. *American Journal of Psychiatry*, 150(2), 188–196.

Hailes, H. P., Ceccolini, C. J., Gutowski, E., & Liang, B. (2020, February 6). Ethical guidelines for social justice in psychology. *Professional Psychology: Research and Practice*. Advance online publication. doi:10.1037/pro0000291

Hammel, G. A., Olkin, R., & Taube, D. O. (1996). Student-educator sex in clinical and counseling psychology doctoral training. *Professional Psychology: Research and Practice*, 27(1), 93–97.

Handelsman, M. M. (1998). Ethics and ethical reasoning. In S. Cullari (Ed.), *Foundations of clinical psychology* (pp. 80–111). Needham Heights, MA: Allyn & Bacon.

Handelsman, M. M. (2001a). Accurate and effective informed consent. In E. R. Welfel & R. E. Ingersoll (Eds.), *The mental health desk reference* (pp. 453–458). New York: Wiley.

Handelsman, M. M. (2001b). Learning to become ethical. In S. Walfish & A. K. Hess (Eds.), *Succeeding in graduate school: The career guide for psychology students* (pp. 189–202). Mahwah, NJ: Lawrence Erlbaum.

Handelsman, M. M. (2017, August 28). Bad justifications for bad behavior [blog post]. https://www.psychologytoday.com/us/blog/the-ethical-professor/201708/bad-justifications-bad-behavior

Handelsman, M. M., Gottlieb, M. C., & Knapp, S. (2005). Training ethical psychologists: An acculturation model. *Professional Psychology: Research and Practice*, 36(1), 59–65.

Handelsman, M. M., Knapp, S., & Gottlieb, M. C. (2009). Positive ethics: Themes and variations. In C. R. Snyder & S. J. Lopez (Eds.), *Oxford handbook of positive psychology* (2nd ed., pp. 105–113). New York: Oxford University Press.

Harrar, W. R., VandeCreek, L., & Knapp, S. (1990). Ethical and legal aspects of clinical supervision. *Professional Psychology: Research and Practice*, 21(1), 37–41.

Harro, B. (2013). The socialization cycle. In M. Adams, W. J. Blumenfeld, C. Castaneda, J. W. Hackman, M. L. Peters, & X. Zuniga (Eds.), *Readings for diversity and social justice* (3rd ed., pp. 45–52). New York: Routledge.

Haynes, R., Corey, G., & Moulton, P. (2003). *Clinical supervision in the helping profession: A practical guide*. Pacific Grove, CA: Brooks/Cole.

Henderson, C. E., Cawyer, C. S., & Watkins, C. E. (1999). A comparison of student and supervisor perceptions of effective practicum supervision. *Clinical Supervisor*, 18(1), 47–74.

Holloway, E. L. (1992). Supervision: A way of learning and teaching. In S. D. Brown & R. W. Lent (Eds.), *Handbook of counseling psychology* (2nd ed., pp. 177–214). New York: Wiley.

Inman, A. G., Hutman, H., Pendse, A., Devdas, L., Luu, L., & Ellis, M. V. (2014). Current trends concerning supervisors, supervisees, and clients in clinical supervision. In C. E. Watkins & D. L. Milne (Eds.), *The Wiley international handbook of clinical supervision* (pp. 65–102). Malden, MA: Wiley-Blackwell.

Jaffee v. Redmond (95–266), 518 U.S. 1 (1996).

Jensen, P. S., Josephson, A. M., & Frey, J. (1989). Informed consent as a framework for treatment: Ethical and therapeutic concerns. *American Journal of Psychotherapy*, 43(3), 378–386.

Jevne, P., & Williams, D. R. (1998). *When dreams don't work: Professional caregivers and burnout*. Amityville, NY: Baywood.

Jordan, A., & Meara, N. (1990). Ethics and the professional practice of psychologists: The role of virtues and principles. *Professional Psychology: Theory and Practice*, 21(2), 106–114.

Jorgenson, L. M., Hirsch, A. B., & Wahl, K. M. (1997). Fiduciary duty and boundaries: Acting in the client's best interest. *Behavioral Sciences & the Law*, 15(1), 49–62.

Ju, A. (2008, May 24). Courage is the most important virtue, says writer and civil rights activist Maya Angelou at Convocation. Cornell Chronicle. https://news.cornell.edu/stories/2008/05/courage-most-important-virtue-maya-angelou-tells-seniors

Kahneman, D. (2011). *Thinking, fast and slow*. New York: Farrar, Straus and Giroux.

Kahneman, D., & Tversky, A. (1973). On the psychology of prediction. *Psychological Review*, 80(4), 237–251.

Kennard, B. D., Stewart, S. M., & Gluck, M. R. (1987). The supervisory relationship: Variables contributing to positive versus negative experiences. *Professional Psychology: Research and Practice*, 18(2), 172–175.

Kilminster, S. M., & Jolly, B. C. (2000). Effective supervision in clinical practice settings: A literature review. *Medical Education*, 34(10), 87–840.

Kitchener, K. S. (2000). *Foundations of ethical practice, research, and teaching in psychology*. Mahwah, NJ: Lawrence Erlbaum.

Kitchener, K. S., & Anderson, S. K. (2011). *Foundations of ethical practice, research, and teaching in psychology and counseling* (2nd ed.). New York: Routledge/Taylor & Francis Group.

Knapp, S. J., Gottlieb, M. C., & Handelsman, M. M. (2015). *Ethical dilemmas in psychotherapy: Positive approaches to decision making*. Washington, DC: American Psychological Association.

Knapp, S. J., VandeCreek, L. D., & Fingerhut, R. (2017). *Practical ethics for psychologists: A positive approach* (3rd ed.). Washington, DC: American Psychological Association.

Kramer, S. A. (1986). The termination process in open-ended psychotherapy: Guidelines for clinical practice. *Psychotherapy*, 23(4), 526–531.

Ladany, N., Ellis, M. V., & Friedlander, M. L. (1999). The supervisory working alliance, trainee self-efficacy, and satisfaction with supervision. *Journal of Counseling & Development*, 77(4), 447–455.

Lambert, M. J., & Barley, D. E. (2002). Psychotherapy relationships that work: Therapist contributions and responsiveness to patients. In J. C. Norcross (Ed.), *Research summary on the therapeutic relationship and psychotherapy outcome. Expectations and preferences* (pp. 17–32). London: Oxford University Press.

Lazarus, A. A. (2007). Restrictive Draconian views must be vigorously challenged. *Professional Psychology: Research and Practice*, 38(4), 405–406.

Lazarus, A. A., & Zur, O. (2002). *Dual relationships and psychotherapy*. New York: Springer.

Liddle, B. J. (2011). Tales from the heart of Dixie: Using white privilege to fight racism. In S. K. Anderson & V. A. Middleton (Eds.), *Explorations in diversity: Examining the complexities of privilege, discrimination, and oppression* (2nd ed., pp. 251–256). New York: Oxford University Press.

Lloyd-Hazlett, J., & Foster, V. A. (2017). Student counselors' moral, intellectual, and professional ethical identity development. *Counseling and Values*, 62(1), 90–105.

Lo, K. (2011). Seeing through another lens. In S. K. Anderson & V. A. Middleton (Eds.), *Explorations in diversity: Examining the complexities of privilege, discrimination, and oppression* (3rd ed., pp. 49–52). New York: Oxford University Press.

Loganbill, C., Hardy, E., & Delworth, U. (1983). Supervision: A conceptual model. *Counseling Psychologist*, 10(1), 3–42.

Loomis, C. (2011). Understanding and experiencing class privilege. In S. K. Anderson & V. A. Middleton (Eds.), *Explorations in diversity: Examining the complexities of privilege, discrimination, and oppression* (2nd ed., pp. 39–47). New York: Oxford University Press.

Lustig, M., & Koester, J. (1999). *Intercultural competence: Interpersonal communication across cultures* (3rd ed.). New York: Addison Wesley Longman.

Maki, D. R., & Bernard, J. M. (2007). The ethics of clinical supervision. In R. R. Cottone & V. M. Tarvydas (Eds.), *Counseling ethics and decision making* (3rd ed., pp. 347–368). Upper Saddle River, NJ: Pearson Merrill Prentice Hall.

Martinez, R. (2000). A model for boundary dilemmas: Ethical decision making in the patient–physician relationship. *Ethical Human Sciences and Services*, 2(1), 43–61.

Martino, C. (2001, August). Secrets of successful supervision: Graduate students' preferences and experiences with effective and ineffective supervision. In J. E. Barnett (Chair), *Secrets of successful supervision—Clinical and ethical issues*. Symposium conducted at the 109th Annual Convention of the American Psychological Association. San Francisco, CA.

McCarthy Veach, P. M., Yoon, E., Miranda, C., MacFarlane, I. M., Ergun, D., & Tuicomepee, A. (2012). Clinical supervisor value conflicts: Low-frequency, but high-impact events. *The Clinical Supervisor*, 31(2), 203–227.

McIntosh, P. (1990, Winter). White privilege: Unpacking the invisible knapsack. *Independent School*, 49(2), 31–36.

McIntosh, P. (2000). White privilege and male privilege: A personal account of coming to see correspondences through work in women's studies. In A. Minas (Ed.), *Gender basics: Feminist perspectives on women and men* (2nd ed., pp. 30–38). Belmont, CA: Wadsworth/Thomas Learning, Inc.

McNamara, M. L., Kangos, K. A., Corp, D. A., Ellis, M. V., & Taylor, E. J. (2017). Narratives of harmful clinical supervision: Synthesis and recommendations. *The Clinical Supervisor*, 36(1), 124–144.

Meara, N., Schmidt, L., & Day, J. (1996). Principles and virtues: A foundation for ethical decisions, policies, and character. *The Counseling Psychologist*, 24(1), 4–77.

Monson, V. E., & Hamilton, N. W. (2010). Entering law students' conceptions of an ethical professional identity and the role of the lawyer in society. *Journal of the Legal Profession*, 35(1), 385–421.

Murray, B. (2012). Informed consent: What must a physician disclose to a patient? *AMA Journal of Ethics*, 14(7), 563–566. doi:10.1001/virtualmentor.2012.14.7.hlaw1-1207

Murray, H. A. (1938). *Explorations in personality*. New York: Oxford University Press.

Myers, D., & Hayes, J. A. (2006). Effects of therapist general self-disclosure and CT disclosure on ratings of the therapist and session. *Psychotherapy*, 43(2), 173–185.

Myers, J. E., Sweeney, T. J., & Witmer, J. M. (2000). The wheel of wellness counseling for wellness: A holistic model. *Journal of Counseling and Development*, 78(3), 251–266.

Nagy, T. F. (2000). *Ethics in plain English*. Washington, DC: American Psychological Association.

National Association of Social Workers. (2017). *Code of ethics of the National Association of Social Workers*. Washington, DC: Author.

O'Donohue, W. T., & Cucciare, M. A. (2008). Introduction. In W. T. O'Donohue & M. A. Cucciare (Eds.), *Terminating psychotherapy: A clinician's guide* (pp. xv–xxvi). New York: Routledge.

O'Reilly, R. (1987). The transfer syndrome. *Canadian Journal of Psychiatry*, 32(8), 674–678.

Owen, J. J., Tao, K., Leach, M. M., & Rodolfa, E. (2011). Clients' perceptions of their psychotherapists' multicultural orientation. *Psychotherapy*, 48(3), 274–282.

Parks, L., & Guay, R. P. (2009). Personality, values, and motivation. *Personality and Individual Differences*, 47(7), 675–684.

Peterson, C., & Seligman, M. E. P. (2004). *Character strengths and virtues: A handbook and classification*. New York: Oxford University Press.

Pettifor, J. L. (2004). Professional ethics across national boundaries. *European Psychologist*, 9(4), 264–272.

Pomerantz, A., & Handelsman, M. M. (2004). Informed consent revisited: An updated written question format. *Professional Psychology: Research and Practice*, 35(2), 201–205.

Pope, K. S., Sonne, J. L., & Greene, B. (2006). *What therapists don't talk about and why*. Washington, DC: American Psychological Association.

Pope, K. S., & Vetter, V. A. (1992). Ethical dilemmas encountered by members of the APA: A national survey. *American Psychologist*, 47(3), 397–411.

Pronin, E., Lin, D. Y., & Ross, L. (2002). The bias blind spot: Perceptions of bias in self versus others. *Personality and Social Psychology Bulletin*, 28(3), 369–381. doi:10.1177/0146167202286008

Reinert, C., & Kowacs, C. (2019). Patient-targeted "googling:" When therapists search for information about their patients online. *Psychodynamic Psychiatry*, 47(1), 27–38. doi:10.1521/pdps.2019.47.1.27

Rest, J. R. (1983). Morality. In J. Flavell & E. Markman (Eds.), In P. Mussen (General Ed.). *Manual of child psychology*. Cognitive development (Vol. IV). New York: Wiley.

Rest, J. R. (1984). Research on moral development: Implications for training counseling psychologists. *Counseling Psychologist*, 12(3), 19–29.

Rest, J. R. (1994). Background: Theory and research. In J. R. Rest & D. Navarez (Eds.), *Moral development in the professions: Psychology and applied ethics* (pp. 1–26). Hillsdale, NJ: Lawrence Erlbaum.

Rice, N. M., & Follette, V. M. (2003). The termination and referral of clients. In W. O'Donohue & K. Ferguson (Eds.), *Handbook of professional ethics for psychologists: Issues, questions, and controversies* (pp. 147–166). Thousand Oaks, CA: Sage.

Rogerson, M. D., Gottlieb, M. C., Handelsman, M. M., Knapp, S., & Younggren, J. (2011). Nonrational processes in ethical decision making. *American Psychologist*, 66(7), 614–623.

Ross, W. D. (1998). *The right and the good*. Oxford: Clarendon Press. Original work published in 1930.

Schwartz, S. H. (1994). Are there universal aspects in the structure and contents of human values? *Journal of Social Issues*, 50(4), 19–45.

Sezer, O., Gino, F., & Bazerman, M. H. (2015). Ethical blind spots: Explaining unintentional unethical behavior. *Current Opinion in Psychology*, 6, 77–81.

Sherry, P. (1991). Ethical issues in the conduct of supervision. *The Counseling Psychologist*, 19(4), 566–585.

Siegel, M. (1979). Privacy, ethics, and confidentiality. *Professional Psychology: Research and Practice*, 10(2), 249–258.

Simon, R. J. (1992). Treatment boundary violations: Clinical, ethical, and legal considerations. *Bulletin of the American Academy of Psychiatry and Law*, 20(3), 269–288.

Skovholt, T. M., & Trotter-Mathison, M. (2016). *Burnout and compassion fatigue prevention and self-care strategies for the helping professions* (3rd ed.). London: Routledge.

Smith, D., & Fitzpatrick, M. (1995). Patient–therapist boundary issues: An integrative review of theory and research. *Professional Psychology: Research and Practice*, 26(5), 499–506.

Spanierman, L. B., Todd, N. R., & Anderson, C. J. (2009). Psychosocial costs of racism to Whites: Understanding patterns among university students. *Journal of Counseling Psychology*, 56(2), 239–252.

Speight, S. L. (2012). An exploration of boundaries and solidarity in counseling relationships. *The Counseling Psychologist*, 40(1), 133–157.

Stoltenberg, C., & Delworth, U. (1987). *Supervising counselors and therapists: A developmental approach*. San Francisco, CA: Jossey Bass.

Sue, D. W., Sue, D., Neville, H. A., & Smith, L. (2019). *Counseling the culturally diverse: Theory and practice* (8th ed.). Hoboken, NJ: Wiley.

Sullivan, T., Martin, W. L., Jr., & Handelsman, M. M. (1993). Practical benefits of an informed consent procedure. *Professional Psychology: Research and Practice*, 24(2), 160–163.

Swift, J. K., & Greenberg, R. P. (2012). Premature discontinuation in adult psychotherapy: A meta-analysis. *Journal of Consulting and Clinical Psychology*, 80(4), 547–559.

Tarasoff v. Regents of the University of California, 529 P.2d 553 (Cal. 1974), 551 P.2d 334, 331 (Cal. 1976).

Tenbrunsel, A., & Messick, D. M. (2004). Ethical fading: The role of self-deception in unethical behavior. *Social Justice Research*, 17(2), 223–236.

Thomas, J. T. (2005). Licensing board complaints: Minimizing the impact on the psychologist's defense and clinical practice. *Professional Psychology: Research and Practice*, 36(4), 426–433.

Trachsel, M., Grosse Holtforth, M., Biller-Andorno, N., & Appelbaum, P. S. (2015). Informed consent for psychotherapy: Still not routine. *The Lancet Psychiatry*, 2(9), 775–777.

Tuason, M. T. (2005). Deprivations and privileges we all have. In S. K. Anderson & V. A. Middleton (Eds.), *Explorations in privilege, oppression and discrimination* (pp. 41–47). Belmont, CA: Thomson Brooks/Cole.

Vasquez, M. J. (1996). Will virtue ethics improve ethical conduct in multicultural settings and interactions? *The Counseling Psychologist*, 24(1), 98–104.

Vasquez, M. J. T. (2007). Sometimes a taco is just a taco! *Professional Psychology: Research and Practice*, 38, 406–407.

Veatch, R. M., & Sollitto, S. (1976). Medical ethics teaching: Report of a national medical school survey. *Journal of the American Medical Association*, 235(10), 1030–1033.

Watkins, C. E. (1995). Psychotherapy supervision in the 1990s: Some observations and reflections. *American Journal of Psychotherapy*, 49(4), 568–581.

Watkins, C. E., Jr., Hook, J. N., DeBlaere, C., Davis, D. E., Van Tongeren, D. R., Owen, J., & Callahan, J. L. (2019). Humility, ruptures, and rupture repair in clinical supervision: A simple conceptual clarification and extension. *The Clinical Supervisor*, 38(2), 281–300.

Welfel, E. R. (2006). *Ethics in counseling and psychotherapy: Standards, research, and emerging issues* (3rd ed.). Belmont, CA: Thomson Brooks/Cole.

Welfel, E. R. (2016). *Ethics in counseling and psychotherapy: Standards, research, and emerging issues* (6th ed.). Boston: Cengage.

Wise, E. H. (2007). Informed consent: Complexities and meanings. *Professional Psychology: Research and Practice*, 38(2), 182–183.

Wulf, J., & Nelson, M. L. (2000). Experienced psychologists' recollections of internship supervision and its contributions to their development. *Clinical Supervisor*, 19(2), 123–145.

Younggren, J. N., & Harris, E. A. (2008). Can you keep a secret? Confidentiality in psychotherapy. *Journal of Clinical Psychology*, 64(5), 589–600.

Zetzer, H. A. (2018). Whiteout: growing out of the problem of white privilege. In S. K. Anderson & V. A. Middleton (Eds.), *Explorations in diversity: Examining the complexities of privilege, discrimination, and oppression* (3rd ed., pp. 9–24). New York: Oxford University Press.

Zuckerman, M. (1979). Attribution of success and failure revisited, or: The motivational bias is alive and well in attribution theory. *Journal of Personality*, 47(2), 245–287.

Zur, O., & Lazarus, A. (2002). Six arguments against dual relationships and their rebuttals. In A. Lazarus & O. Zur (Eds.), *Dual relationships and psychotherapy* (pp. 3–24). New York: Springer.

Author Index

Subject Index

Note: Page numbers with italic *f* and *t* denote figures and tables